Endometriosis

Endometriosis

Natural and medical solutions

Kaz Cooke
& Ruth Trickey

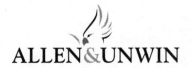

ALLEN&UNWIN

Thanks to Gemma Ridgeway-Faye for editing assistance on this series.

Allen & Unwin
83 Alexander Street
Crows Nest NSW 2065
Australia
Phone: (61 2) 8425 0100
Fax: (61 2) 9906 2218
Email: info@allenandunwin.com
Web: www.allenandunwin.com

National Library of Australia
Cataloguing-in-Publication entry:

Cooke, Kaz, 1962- .
    Endometriosis : natural and medical solutions.

    Includes index.
    ISBN 1 86508 761 0.

    1. Endometriosis. 2. Endometriosis - Treatment. 3.
    Endometriosis - Alternative treatment. I. Trickey, Ruth,
    1953- . II. Title.

618.1

Cover and text design by Dianna Wells Design
Set in 12/14 pt MrsEavesRoman by Bookhouse, Sydney
Printed in Australia by McPherson's Printing Group

10 9 8 7 6 5 4 3 2

Contents

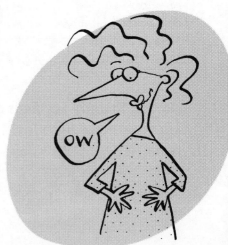

ABOUT THE AUTHORS

Ruth Trickey is a herbalist with a nursing and midwifery background. She specialises in the application of Chinese and Western herbal treatments of women's health problems. She runs the Melbourne Holistic Health Group in Melbourne, and treats many patients in conjunction with their doctors and surgeons. Ruth is the author of *Women, Hormones and the Menstrual Cycle*, and a frequent lecturer and guest speaker in Australia, New Zealand, Europe and North America.

Kaz Cooke is a cartoonist and author with a history of severe endometriosis. She is the author of *Real Gorgeous: the Truth About Body and Beauty*; *Up the Duff: the Real Guide to Pregnancy*; *Living With Crazy Buttocks*; a children's book called *The Terrible Underpants* and the satirical *Little Book of . . .* series, encompassing Stress, Dumb Feng Shui, Household Madness, Beauty, and Diet and Exercise.

Most of the information in this small book is edited and updated from the text of *Women's Trouble*, by the same authors, also published by Allen & Unwin. A full list of acknowledgements and footnotes is published in *Women's Trouble*. Also in this series of small books on women's health: *Menopause* and *Problem Periods*.

All advice given in this book is general and not intended to be used instead of professional medical advice. Any of the advice herein should be undertaken only after consultation with your doctor and natural therapies practitioner. Each person in your advice team must be aware of all drugs, herbs and other treatments you are undergoing. It is not safe to self-diagnose, or self-prescribe with either herbs or drugs. Individual and tailored treatments can only be obtained from your own practitioners.

Intro

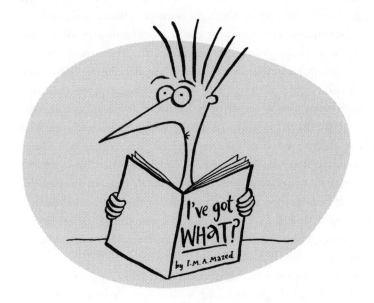

Endometriosis is a mystery. No-one knows for sure why it happens, but plenty of people will tell you their pet theory—whether you're interested or not—such as 'having a baby cures it' (not necessarily true) or 'it means you'll be infertile' (not necessarily true) and 'you'll be right; my cousin Shazza had endo and now she's got nine kids' (not necessarily true; and someone send Shazza a medal).

It's very hard to prevent 'endo' or its close relative, adenomyosis, because there's a mixed bag of theories about why it happens, and who's most likely to get it. It's hard to diagnose because it causes heaps of different symptoms—from period pain and heavy periods to painful sex and irritable bowel syndrome—and because some doctors assume the pain is ordinary period pain which will 'settle down', especially in younger women. Many women have experienced endo symptoms for years before they have their problem correctly diagnosed, often in their late twenties or early thirties. Others are now being diagnosed in their teenage years, and face unique problems dealing with pain and even surgery before they're all grown up.

Because of ignorance about endo, many women who are diagnosed don't know whether to expect to change their diet or have a hysterectomy (the two ends of the treatment spectrum). Because so many women have endo, and there is money to be made from the medical industry, we can expect a steady stream of new drugs, other treatments, surgical innovations and maybe even a cure one day.

You can't predict the future, and you can't even predict you will be diagnosed with endo even if you have some of the problems on the list of symptoms (page 11). So here's some advice: if you can afford it, take out private health insurance that covers surgery and natural therapies right now, before you investigate anything further. If you can't afford it, fear not, because if you need surgical treatment you can get it in the public system. But you may have to be on a waiting list, and may not be able to choose the surgeon. And some herbal and natural therapies treatments are expensive.

Endometriosis can be very tricky to treat—a process of trial and error is often unavoidable because endo is

 2

different in each person. Decisions about treatment are complex and sometimes the best course of action is anybody's guess. Despite the anecdotal Shazza factor, predictions about future fertility are almost impossible.

As a matter of fact, if your endo doctor says there is nothing to be done, or 'My dear girlie, I know exactly what will cure you, and I understand exactly the extent of your endo without looking inside you and I'll have you cured in a jiffy and give you buckets of babies', then run away. Also run right away if your natural health practitioner says, 'I have a secret theory about endo that nobody else knows about. It happens because you are dehydrated/not eating enough essence of moose antler/not comfortable with your feminine side (etc).'

Sometimes family and friends don't understand the problem. 'It's just a bit of period pain'; 'get over it'; 'pull yourself together'. Endo pain is invisible, not like a broken arm. It can go on for years causing emotional damage to you and your relationships. But you can get a hold of this thing and deal with it from many angles. You can take control and stop it controlling you. In this book, we talk about the medical, natural therapies and self care options for treating all the aspects of endo, including pain; premenstrual syndrome symptoms (PMS); heavy periods; and depression.

So, it's time for just one last anxious panic before you start getting everything under control and get back in the metaphorical driver's seat of your own health. (It is a very snazzy metaphorical sports coupé with metaphorical 6-CD stacker full of allegorical Aretha Franklin.) Right, just before you pull yourself together, go and get a pillow, press your face into it and have a long, last scream of frustration.

Aaaaaaaaarrrrrggggghhhh!!! Okay. It's all uphill from here. Time to find some collaborators.

Having endo is difficult enough without dealing with the smug or narrow-minded shockers out there. ('Don't go to a doctor—they don't know anything'; 'Don't even think about natural therapies, they're all feral hippies with no training'.) You may well find that a combination of medical and natural solutions works best for you. Find some practitioners who say, 'I have a lot of experience in the field, this is my specialty. I can make educated guesses and try various things and we'll work together to find the best treatment for you.'

It's true that having endo can make you feel like a 'victim' in a body that had betrayed you. But take heart and start to take control of your health. Lots of people do get over endo, lots of other people will always have it but manage the pain, and there's a lot we do know and that might help. This is the condition that led to the meeting of your authors—Kaz took her endo along to see Ruth, and believe us when we say we've really been through it!

Please remember that as long as your doctor and natural therapist can work together, there's no need to choose one method of treatment over the other, exclusively. You may need a mix of surgery, drug and natural treatments to control your condition. Try to keep open-minded about what might help you. (Not too open-minded. Alien space rays generally don't work, we've found.)

Need to find a new doctor and/or natural therapist? A good place to start is a support group in your area, which you can find by seeing the list on page 155. In the meantime, here's the inside story on endometriosis:

WHAT IS IT?

Normally, a layer of endometrium which lines the inside of the uterus is expelled, as period 'blood', during each period. When you've got endometriosis, some of this endometrial tissue starts to grow elsewhere in the body, instead. Usually the endometrium doesn't travel very far, and is found mostly somewhere within the pelvic region.

ENDOMETRIOSIS can be on the ovaries, the Fallopian tubes, the outside wall of the uterus, the uterine or ovarian ligaments, the bowel, the ureters, the tube leading from the kidney to the bladder, or the bladder itself, or the Pouch of Douglas which is the space between the uterus and the bowel. It can be on the vagina, cervix or vulva. Some people have even found it on their eyelids and navel and other distant places. It's pesky stuff. The name endometriosis comes from the ancient Greek for within, *endon*, and the word for uterus, *metra*. The *osis* bit on the end is Greek for process, in this case, a disease process. We'll just call it endo.

ADENOMYOSIS is more specific: endometrium growing between the fibres of the muscular wall of the uterus. (*Adeno* is ancient Greek for glandular.) One of the main problems with endo is that the endometrial cells in the wrong place keep trying to act like they're in the uterus getting ready in case an egg wants to implant. So

5

each month they grow, and then bleed away again, basically causing new implants and getting bigger. If you could see the endometrial implants, they would look like bluish or reddish patches or bubbles. On the ovaries, they look like cysts of darkened brown blood—and doctors often call them 'chocolate cysts' although how they can face a Mars Bar after that is a mystery, too.

Endo causes pain because these 'cysts' or 'implants' are growing in the wrong place and causing pressure and organs to stick together which shouldn't stick together (called 'adhesions'), and blockages where they shouldn't be, all mostly in the pelvis and on all the most delicate reproductive gear we've got, like Fallopian tubes, and that's why it can lead to infertility. But having endo doesn't mean you're automatically infertile, because it depends on how much damage has been done to which parts and how sneaky the body can be to get around it.

Endo is usually diagnosed after a long search for what's causing pain or difficulty in getting pregnant. It is the cause of up to 80 per cent of pelvic pain or infertility. Endo also tends to come back: about half of all women with endo develop it again within five years of successful treatment.

WHO HAS IT?

Most estimates suggest that between 1 and 10 per cent of women have endo. But these might be conservative estimates because usually only women who have pain or infertility have investigative surgery—which is the only foolproof way to diagnose it. Doctors doing surgery for other reasons who also have a look round for endo find that more like 15–20 per cent of women have it. The trick is that a lot of women don't have any trouble or pain from their endo and never even know it's there.

Some researchers believe there are various types of endo, some not as severe as others, because only some women develop endometriosis that causes pain or infertility. Other researchers think it's your individual health which determines the extent of your endo symptoms. Women with a good immune system and inflammatory responses may prevent the endo getting a hold in their bodies without even knowing it.

WHAT DOES IT DO?

Cysts and deposits

About 60 per cent of women with endo develop cysts in the ovaries (ovarian cysts) which vary from microscopic spots to a growth the size of a tennis ball. When small, the endo growths look a bit like blood blisters and are reddish-blue, or brown if the blood is old. Both ovaries are usually affected. The ovary usually tries to contain the growth of the endometrial tissue by creating a capsule around it, and a cyst is formed. These cysts are either called endometriomas, 'chocolate cysts' or endometrial cysts, and are filled by endometrial blood shed at each period.

Even when small, these cysts can rupture and spill their contents within the pelvis area. Unruptured cysts keep growing within their thickened capsule. The endo tissue inside still responds to hormonal change in the same way as normal endometrium and bleeds with each period, causing the cysts to get bigger every month. Eventually the blood becomes thick, sticky and dark brown.

There may be increasing pain as the cysts become larger and press on other organs, blood vessels and nerves.

Occasionally, cysts wither away because the internal pressure deprives the cyst of a blood supply and it atrophies. Former atrophied cysts can be identified by the little white scars they leave on the ovarian tissue. Alternatively, the cyst may grow painlessly, but the risk of rupture multiplies as the months go by. When really large cysts rupture, they cause symptoms of acute abdominal pain and shock which has to be treated by immediate surgery. This rush-to-the-hospital situation is relatively rare because cysts almost always rupture before they get big, or are diagnosed way before they can get out of hand.

Even a very small amount of the blood shed during this kind of rupture will cause inflammation and pain. These common, smaller cyst ruptures usually happen during or just after a period, and are a prime suspect in causing endo pain.

Endo can be anywhere in the pelvis as well as the ovaries. Common endo sites are the previously mentioned and weirdly named Pouch of Douglas, which sits between the uterus and the bowel; the uterine ligaments, which are like tent-ropes which tether the uterus in the right place; and the peritoneum, a clingfilm-like layer which is draped over the outside surfaces of all your pelvic organs, including the ovaries. As the endo gets worse, the implants tend to merge together and form larger islands of endometrial implants.

Adhesions

For some months the endo tissue will usually 'menstruate' at each period, but as the disease advances, scar tissue develops as the body tries to isolate the irritating intruder and 'wall off' the problem area. Lumps form over the tissues and organs that have become invaded by the endometrial implants: the adhesions (scar tissue). Adhesions usually solidify over time and become thick and fibrous. (Adhesions can also be caused by internal healing after a surgical operation.)

If the endo just keeps getting worse, the body makes more and more adhesions. The tissue and organs near the endo get progressively covered and plastered down by scar tissue. Eventually the pelvic organs can become one large immoveable mass. Any movement of these constricted organs can cause pain or discomfort, for example, during sex or an examination by a doctor, or when having a poo.

Emotional side effects

Severe or seemingly uncontrollable pain, the problems with sex, the feeling that the body is betraying you, worries about the present and the future, confusion about the best way to treat the problem, the possible problems with fertility associated with damage caused by endometrial implants: all these can cause depression and bewilderment. Whether diagnosed or undiagnosed, endometriosis can prompt a whole range of feelings related to confusion and despair. Hormone imbalances, too, will contribute to mood swings.

WHAT CAUSES IT?

Almost everyone who gets endo gets it when they are producing oestrogen and menstruating regularly. But other factors must be needed to cause endo, or we'd all have it. The fact is, doctors don't know yet what causes endo but there are some factors which are prime suspects—alone or perhaps together:

- too much oestrogen;
- a cellular change to the tissue covering the uterine wall;
- a retrograde flow of period blood backwards through the Fallopian tubes and out into the pelvis;
- an imbalance of hormone-like properties called prostaglandins and leukotrienes (more of these later) can cause problems with ovulation, fertilisation, embryo development, and the function of the Fallopian tube. The wrong levels of prostaglandins and leukotrienes can also make the period pain worse;
- a problem with the immune system that lets the endo deposits get out of hand.

SYMPTOMS

Adenomyosis and (especially) endometriosis have wildly varying symptoms ranging from really severe and near constant pain, dragging feelings in the pelvis, very painful penetrative sex, abnormal bleeding, shocking premenstrual tension, and infertility, all the way down to not a single symptom in sight. The most common endo symptoms are:

- really bad period pain;
- difficulty getting pregnant;
- pain during sex, particularly during penetration;
- pain getting worse toward the end of periods;
- pain before periods and at ovulation;
- pelvic pain on one side;
- irritable bowel syndrome—swinging between constipation and diarrhoea, with wind problems;
- pain when pooing;
- any of the above symptoms worse during or associated with the period;
- PMS symptoms;
- heavy periods;
- a sister or mother with endo.

If you've got all these symptoms you've probably hit the endo jackpot. (You may have endo even if you don't have all of the symptoms.) Getting your first period at an early age, long periods (more than seven days) and heavy periods are associated with an increased risk of endo. (Long and irregular breaks between periods are associated with a lowered risk.) If you describe all these symptoms and related factors and your doctor says, 'It's just a slight head cold' or 'Nothing to worry about there, missy' make sure you're out of that office in in two seconds flat. Some of us can spend years getting a diagnosis. Many GPs are much better informed about endo now, but a few are not. If you suspect endo, make sure you get a referral to a specialist—in this case, a gynaecologist at the very least.

And make sure you are not diagnosed by a natural therapist. Even if you have all or most of the above symptoms, any practitioner can only give you a presumed diagnosis—you will almost certainly need a medical diagnosis, such as a laparoscopy, before you can be certain that you have endo. Of course a natural therapist can help you with any of the above symptoms—but it's very important to know what the underlying problem is.

Pain

Unless you move in long-distance swimming circles, any mysterious mention of 'the cramps' is always assumed to be about period pain. So many of us get period pain that it could be called usual—but that doesn't make it normal. Lots of people, some of them doctors and natural therapists, think that a bit of period pain is normal. Patients get used to hearing stuff like, 'Grin and bear it', that hoary old chestnut 'It will be better once you have a baby' and even 'It's just part of being a woman.' Bollocks. It's not something you should put up with, or expect as part of your womanly life. (You're a woman now, and you will have period pain and an automatic instinct for the correct hat for every occasion? Not very scientific.)

The thing is, a bit of period pain is usual, but just because it's common, doesn't mean that it's normal or nothing to worry about. The most important thing about persistent period pain is to find out what's causing it. If your treatments for the pain aren't working, get investigative—it could be a warning from your body about something serious.

The two questions to ask about period pain are: 'Does it bother you enough to want/need to do something about it?' If not, you are excused. Go and sit in the corner and

12

try on some hats until the end of this section. If your period pain is bad enough to make you do something about it, here's another question: 'Are you happy with the treatments you are using?' If not, read on. It may be well worth your while: after all, on average you have 12 or 13 periods a year, and if you get pain for two or three days, that adds up to a month of pain each year: yikes.

Doctors often call period pain dysmenorrhoea. It sounds rather disgusting, but is basically just ancient Greek for painful periods: *dys* meaning difficulty with, and *menorrhoea* meaning to do with menstruation. It's pronounced dis-men-oh-rear. Dysmenorrhoea is a symptom, not a disease—so the first aspect of any successful treatment is to find out why you're getting pain.

Period pain falls into two major categories:

- The uterine muscle is behaving abnormally and causing cramps, but is otherwise healthy. This is called naughty uterus. No, it's actually called primary dysmenorrhoea. (Primary dysmenorrhoea is sometimes also called functional dysmenorrhoea. Are they deliberately trying to confuse us or just SHOWING OFF?)

- A disease of an organ or organs which has pain as one of its symptoms. This is called secondary dysmenorrhoea. Common causes of secondary dysmenorrhoea include endometriosis and pelvic inflammatory disease (PID). But sometimes primary dysmenorrhoea can cause really bad pain and secondary dysmenorrhoea is not so bad—that is, really bad pain doesn't automatically mean you have a disease—in fact in some cases disease doesn't cause pain. PID, for example, is often called a 'silent' disease because in many cases you don't even know you've got it until you're being tested for infertility.

How does it hurt? Let me count the ways
You name it. Period pain can vary dramatically from person to person, and even from period to period. Some have severe pain that feels sharp, or maybe dull. Others have pain that comes in fits and starts. The most common description of period pain is a continual, dull, 'back-ground' ache or sense of heaviness (someone came over all Greek and called it congestive dysmenorrhoea), also accompanied by episodes of cramping pain (spasmodic dysmenorrhoea).

The pain is usually central and under the navel. Sometimes a heavy aching pain extends to the groin, the back, and down the thighs. Most often, the pain that starts before you see the first blood of the period is congestive and aching. Sometimes this sort of pain is accompanied by a heavy dull sense of dragging in the vagina or a sense of fullness in the bowel. This is the feeling often described as though 'everything will fall out'. (You'll be relieved to know it never does.)

Most often, though, the pain starts with the first blood of the period and intensifies as the flow becomes heavier, or when clots are in the period blood. Usually the spas-modic, crampy-type pain is the shortest part of the pain but it feels the worst. During the period, the pain can become sharper, more crampy. For some women, the pain is severe enough to cause fainting, vomiting and diarrhoea.

All that contracting of the uterus can annoy the neighbours—and the bowel is just next door. The bowel tends to be affected by hormone changes too. Many women become constipated before their period and this can exacerbate the sense of fullness and heaviness felt with congestive period pain. Irritable bowel syndrome aggravates period pain and is aggravated by it. The bowel and uterus share a similar nerve supply and when either organ is in spasm, the other will spasm in sympathy.

Period pain usually only happens in a cycle that you have ovulated in, and period pain often only starts in earnest about two years after the first-ever period, when ovulation has become regular. That's why an occasional period can be surprisingly pain-free—maybe you didn't ovulate in that cycle.

There's no relationship between the severity of endo and the severity of the pain. There seems to be no rhyme or reason (why would there be a rhyme? Menstrual pain poetry—there's a genre to avoid if you're looking for a laugh) about the kind of pain, when it comes, or how bad it gets. About one-third of women with endo have no pain.

Many women report pain during sex or during bowel movements. There might be random pain throughout the month; at ovulation; before, during or after the period; or all the time. The symptoms are all over the shop. Get on to a doctor to investigate any strong pain before a period, pain which is only on one side of the body or pelvic pain that doesn't seem related to your period. But any pain—associated with endo or not—which is worrying or interfering with your life needs investigation and treatment.

Symptoms of 'pelvic discomfort', heaviness, or mild pain during a period are often fixed by eating well, exercising regularly and stress reduction. Stronger, crampy pain can also be helped by specific diet and lifestyle changes.

When to see the doctor

- You have some of the symptoms of endo listed on page 11.
- Your period pain changes in some way or you get period pain for the first time.
- The pain is interfering with your life.
- Pain is on one side and/or radiating (spreading to the thigh or another area).
- You have pain at the time of your period that is not like your usual period pain, and there's any possibility you might be pregnant (even if you are on the Pill), especially if accompanied by dizziness or back pain (this could be an ectopic pregnancy, which is a medical emergency).
- Your usual ways of controlling the pain don't seem to work any more.
- New symptoms accompany the pain, for example, vomiting, diarrhoea, or feeling faint.
- The pain gets worse towards the end of the period.
- Pain is aggravated by pressure, bowel motions or sex.
- A fever or discharge accompanies the pain.

Premenstrual syndrome (PMS)

Natural therapists often treat PMS at the same time as treating endo, because if you have endo you probably also have symptoms of PMS including anxiety, mood swings, bloating, breast soreness, constipation, food cravings, and headaches. (Interestingly, all women with endo are strikingly beautiful. Alright, sure we made that bit up, but it did cheer you up for a minute there, didn't it?)

We mightn't know exactly what causes PMS, but we know how it makes us feel. A rather ostentatious 150 different symptoms have been recorded. Luckily, no-one gets all of them at once. Most women have their own little collection of regular PMS symptoms, with the occasional extra one. Symptoms might also change after a major biological event—such as childbirth or illness—and you tend to develop different types of symptoms as you approach menopause. Premenstrual headaches, for example, can become more common. But it is the timing that tells whether you have PMS. There should be no symptoms in the week after the period, but symptoms appearing at any time in the two weeks before a period, and then declining when the period starts.

Most common problems of PMS
- abdominal distension, bloating and discomfort
- breast swelling, pain, discomfort and/or painful, benign breast lumps
- headaches
- abnormal appetite, craving for sweet foods, alcohol and/or fatty foods

17

- fatigue and weakness
- weight gain of more than 2 kilos
- fluid retention
- premenstrual acne
- joint pains and/or backache
- pelvic discomfort or pain
- increased incidence of upper respiratory tract infections, including sinusitis and recurrent colds
- premenstrual genital herpes outbreaks, recurrent vaginal thrush and/or other infections
- change in bowel habit
- palpitations
- dizziness or fainting
- changed sex drive: either you get quite startlingly raunchy suddenly, or go off the very idea of a half-naked fireman (or whatever else takes your fancy)

Most common emotional and mental symptoms

- nervous tension
- mood swings
- tearfulness
- forgetfulness
- anxiety
- aggression
- irritability
- confusion
- insomnia
- depression
- lack of concentration

Natural therapists often break down PMS into several sub-groups for treatment—there's more on that in the Natural Therapy Solutions chapter.

Period flow

The flow of period blood—endometrium—is characteristically slow to start and may be thick and brown to black and tarry at first. Irregular cycles, spotting, and/or midcycle bleeding are also recognisable associations.

Heavy periods

Most women with endo, but not all of them, have a short menstrual cycle and heavy periods.

A mix of symptoms

Keep track of all your symptoms by keeping a menstrual diary—you can use the one below, enlarge it on a photocopier and keep it folded and taped inside your diary. Note the days of your period by circling them, and then add other symptoms in code such as the nature of blood flow (R for red, B for brown, C for clots); pain (CP for cramps, V for vomiting caused by pain, BP for bowel pain when poohing, CT for constipation, and PMS symptoms such as UMD (unspecific morbid dread) and MVS (mad, vile screaming) etc. (Don't forget to keep the key to your code so you can decipher it!) This menstrual diary will help your practitioners make an educated guess at your diagnosis.

DIAGNOSIS

By the time you're reading this book it could be too late to join a private health fund so you don't have to wait for a public operation. But before you get a diagnosis, it

PERIOD SYMPTOMS DIARY: Record the relevant coded number to describe your bleeding and symptoms.

BLEEDING: 0—none 1—slight 2—moderate 3—heavy 4—heavy and clots
SYMPTOMS: 0—none 1—mild; does not interfere with activities 2—moderate; interferes with activities 3—severe; disabling; unable to function

Day of cycle	1	2	3	4	5	6	7	8	9	10	11	12	13	14	15	16	17	18	19	20	21	22	23	24	25	26	27	28	29	30	31	32	33	34	35	36
DATE																																				
BLEEDING																																				
PMS-A SYMPTOMS:																																				
Nervous tension																																				
Mood swings																																				
Irritability																																				
Anxiety																																				
PMS-H SYMPTOMS:																																				
Weight gain																																				
Swelling of extremities																																				
Breast tenderness																																				
Abdominal bloating																																				
PMS-C SYMPTOMS:																																				
Headache																																				
Craving for sweets																																				
Increased appetite																																				
Heart pounding																																				
Fatigue																																				
Dizziness or faintness																																				
PMS-D SYMPTOMS:																																				
Depression																																				
Forgetfulness																																				
Crying																																				
Confusion																																				
Insomnia																																				
PMS-P SYMPTOMS:																																				
Pain																																				
Cramps																																				
Backache																																				
General aches/pain																																				

You can photocopy this diary to use indefinitely.

might be worth getting private health insurance, if you can afford it . . . this will give you more choices. If you don't have private health insurance don't worry—you can still get good treatment for endo if you need it. The main advantages of insurance are rebates for natural therapy treatments, no waiting list for surgery, and being able to choose the surgeon. Check carefully what your fund covers.

Some symptoms you describe may indicate the need for a pelvic examination. The doctor will feel for the pelvic organs and whether they're moving freely or have likely 'adhesions', when cysts or scar tissue has stuck the organs together.

It is usual to be referred for an ultrasound examination or look-around laparoscopy surgery because these are the only ways to definitely diagnose endometriosis.

Ultrasound

An ultrasound for endometriosis or adenomyosis is performed with the same equipment that's used during pregnancy to get an image of the foetus. You will be lying down for the procedure. Either the ultrasound operator will slide a little probe like a computer mouse around on the outside of your bare stomach, or if that won't get a good enough view, they will put a probe inside the vagina. The probe is usually shaped like a smooth pen with a small bulb shape on one end. It's not too big, and may be slightly uncomfortable when they move it around slightly.

The image is projected on a small screen. The ultrasound operator will be able to explain to you what is being seen—otherwise, you're thinking the TV's gone on the blink or something and they're going, 'Ye Gads! It's an ovarian follicle!' (That's a 'casing' where an egg comes from.)

Ultrasound imaging will not reveal endo in the pelvic cavity, but it can usually be relied on for an operator to see adenomyosis or endometriosis cysts in the ovaries. Endo cysts, being made of thickened, dense blood, appear on the ultrasound monitor as darker shapes than other fluid-filled cysts. Other areas of endometriosis, being smaller and less dense, will not show on an ultrasound.

Laparoscopy

A surgical laparoscopy procedure under general anaesthetic is the only way that a diagnosis of endometriosis can be absolutely confirmed. The operation is usually known as a 'look-see' when any major gynaecological problem is suspected, but often, if endo is found, it will be treated at the same time. For this reason it should always be performed by a surgeon who is also skilled in treating endo. (For all the detailed info on laparoscopy and other surgery, see the surgery section in the Medical Solutions chapter.)

TREATMENT

This book outlines the medical, herbal and self care treatments for endo. A mix of treatments is almost always the best solution. To borrow a phrase from Malcolm X, who was speaking about eradicating racism, when asked about his methods: 'by whatever means necessary'.

Medical Solutions

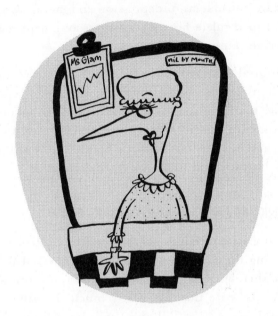

Drug treatment for endo usually aims to do one or several of these things:

- reduce or stop periods, creating a continual pregnancy-like state, on the basis that if there is no endometrium there can be no new endometriosis (continuous doses of the Pill, as well as the progestogens Provera and Danazol);
- reduce the volume of the period flow (the Pill and progestogens);

- cause a temporary menopausal state (the GnRH agonist range of drugs);
- regulate pain (prostaglandins inhibiting drugs, some other painkillers, as well as the Pill);
- address problems of depression and mood swings (the Pill to regulate hormone swings; anti-depressants of various kinds).

Surgical treatment of endo usually aims to remove any adhesions or cysts caused by endo, and try to repair any damage to organs such as the ovaries and Fallopian tubes, if fertility is a priority for you. In extremely chronic severe cases, and as a very last resort, a hysterectomy will put the most dramatic end to the menstrual cycle.

SHRINKING ENDO AND REDUCING FLOW

Several classes of drugs can be used to control endo by shrinking the growth of both the endometrial lining as well as shrinking the endometriosis; or by creating a pregnancy-like state that has pretty much the same result. These drugs are the Pill and the progestogens. A more drastic way of shrinking endo is to use the drugs that can cause a menopause-like state—the GnRH agonists.

The Pill
The Pill is used when women have endometriosis for lots of different reasons. Taking the Pill as commonly prescribed for contraception (21 days on, 7 days off) reduces the amount of period blood and this lowers the risk of developing more endometriosis. It usually reduces

 24

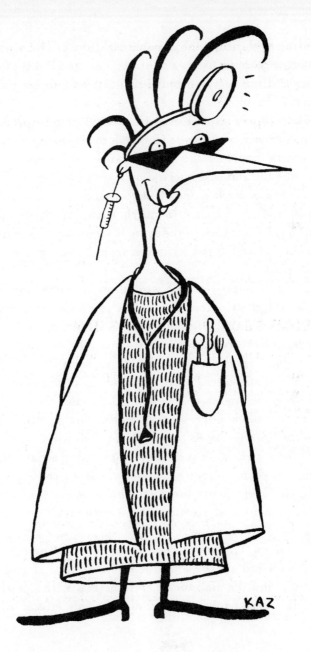

I'm afraid you've got myxomatosis

bleeding by thinning the endometrial lining. This means that apart from its use as a contraceptive, the Pill is often prescribed for heavy periods whether a woman has endo or not.

The Pill can also be used for period pain, especially when you need a contraceptive as well, or if prostaglandins-inhibitors like Naprosyn or Ponstan haven't worked for you. The Pill improves period pain about 90 per cent of the time because it stops ovulation and holds down the prostaglandins which cause muscle spasm. Shrinking the endo also lessens pain by reducing the amount of bleeding into cysts as well as the irritation from bleeding into the pelvic cavity.

The Pill improves PMS symptoms in some women, has no effect in others and makes some women worse. The Pill's control of some women's PMS is probably because it stops ovulation and balances the hormones.

In some severe cases of repeat endo, a doctor will suggest you stay on a Pill with a steady dose of oestrogen and progesterone each day—that is, the dose of the Pill will not mimic a 'normal' cycle, but suppress it. In these cases the Pill will be taken every day, indefinitely, with no break for a 'period' so there will be no endometrial blood going anywhere, because the body is not producing it while you keep taking the Pill. This basically puts your body into a pretend pregnancy state: without all the other symptoms of pregnancy.

The latest Pills have much lower levels of oestrogen which can reduce the amount of both normal endo-metrium and the amount of endometriosis. If it works, the Pill is better for endo, because the side effects from other drugs are much more serious. For example, the GnRH agonists can decrease bone density, while the progesterones are likely to cause mood changes amongst other things. However, the Pill is not as effective for advanced endometriosis and is not suitable for women who want to get pregnant (der). Also, some women who have endo and use the Pill may have trouble getting pregnant when they stop. Others have no problem.

Good points about the Pill
If taken properly, the Pill is probably the most effective contraception aside from not letting sperm anywhere near you. Some other good effects may include reduced rates of ovarian and endometrial cancer, benign breast disease (not breast cancer), benign ovarian cysts, pelvic inflammatory disease, period pain, heavy periods and anaemia. Today's low-dose Pills are much safer than the earlier Pills which had much higher doses of hormones.

Bad points about the Pill
Taking the Pill to combat endo is obviously a fairly hopeless solution if you want to get pregnant. As well, in one study, most women had a return of symptoms within six months of stopping the Pill. The less jolly side effects of the Pill can include blood clots, stroke, and heart attack, especially for smokers. It can cause period changes such as breakthrough bleeding or spotting, and some women experience androgenic blokey hormone effects, including the weight gain and acne which are associated with the progestogen (synthetic progesterone) in the Pill.

A number of women develop long-term loss of periods

after coming off the Pill—estimated to be about 1 per cent after the first year. Some women on the Pill also report an increase in mood swings, depression and loss of interest in sex. These symptoms are more common in the first couple of months of taking the Pill and may go away after that. Doctors usually advise taking one Pill for two months before trying a new brand of Pill which might have fewer side effects for you. Mood changes caused by the Pill are usually related to the progesterones and trying Pills with a different level of this hormone or a Pill where the hormone levels don't change through the months can help. Check for other causes of depression as well—it may not be the Pill.

Warnings in the MIMS and PP Guide (medical books which describe what drugs should be prescribed for, what the drugs do, and when they shouldn't be used) say that periods become lighter and that blood iron levels increase but that oestrogen can make fibroids get bigger (fibroids are benign cysts, usually attached to ovaries or the uterus) which can be associated with heavy bleeding. If you have fibroids and you want to take the Pill, talk to a specialist gynaecologist.

The Pill can cause increased pigmentation of the skin which is known as chloasma or melasma. This usually shows up in patchy, light brown areas on a pale-skinned face and becomes much darker with exposure to the sun. It's not so noticeable on darker skin. It is probably caused by oestrogen—it sometimes also happens in pregnancy, or in women with high oestrogen levels. Stopping the Pill does not necessarily mean that it will go away completely, although it does tend to fade. Use high protection sun screen religiously, and you may lighten the pigmentation with safe skin creams or 'peels' that contain glycolic acid. Doctors sometimes recommend creams containing hydro-quinone or acne medication.

Different types of the Pill and endo

There are heaps of different types of oral contraceptive pills, including Pills with variable oestrogen and progestogen levels (Triphasil and Triquilar), or those with the same levels throughout the cycle (Brevinor, Microgynon). Some also contain androgen-blocking agents (Diane) and are used for acne and excessive male-pattern hair growth; some are progestogen-only Pills (the mini Pills such as Micronor and Microlut). A lot of factors need to be considered when prescribing the Pill. Each different brand or type of Pill can have its own effects on individuals. It's best that a specific brand of Pill is prescribed for you by a gynaecologist who is a specialist in your problem, whether it's PMS or endometriosis. Support groups, listed at the back of the book, will have lists of specialist doctors or clinics you can contact.

Researchers investigating the Pill have come up with some conflicting results about how the Pill might affect endo. Some studies report an increased risk, others a reduced risk, and still others no change. Helpful, isn't it? In another study of more than 17 000 women, the incidence of endo was lower in women currently using the Pill, and higher in former Pill users, compared with women who have never taken the Pill.

Here's how the Pill might influence the risk of endo: the extra oestrogen could increase the risk (although the amount of oestrogen in Pills has been dropping steadily for 30 years); the extra progesterone might decrease risk; and the lighter periods experienced on the Pill might cut out some retrograde flow.

(Incidentally, intra-uterine devices (IUDs) have been linked with an increased incidence of endometriosis, possibly because they encourage retrograde flow and alter prostaglandin levels.)

Other things to take while on the Pill

We'll take a short detour from the medical business to recommend some natural therapies to help with side effects of the Pill:

- The Pill influences a number of nutrients. You'll need more of vitamins B2, B3, B6, folic acid and zinc, but less iron because of the smaller blood loss at the period. If you are on the Pill, a daily B-group vitamin is a good idea, especially one with a B6 level of between 25 and 50 milligrams. (You may be prescribed a larger daily dose.) This may also help with depression and mood changes associated with the Pill.

- Herbal diuretics, especially dandelion leaf tea, can help with fluid retention symptoms. One or two teaspoons a cup, twice daily (not before bed) is the usual dose. Vegetable juices with parsley and celery can also have a diuretic effect, and there are herbal diuretic tablets. Beware of diuretic drugs which can strip the body of potassium. Cut down on salt in food.

- Many women find that evening primrose oil (between 1 and 3 grams a day) is useful for many of the symptoms, such as fluid retention, that they experience

 30

while taking the Pill. Diet can also be altered to take in more essential fatty acids. (See page 120.)

- The blood copper level increases when women are on the Pill and may be partly responsible for the mood changes. High copper levels can lead to a zinc deficiency and zinc supplements may be needed, especially by vegetarians and vegans. A zinc information page is included on page 138. The recommended daily intake of zinc for women while on the Pill is 15-20 milligrams a day.

- Women who smoke and take the Pill can take 250 IU of vitamin E every day to reduce the risk of blood clot formation (but usually not if you have a pre-existing heart condition or high blood pressure). But quite frankly, you are taking a helluva risk smoking while on the Pill. Even women in their twenties and early thirties can have strokes.

- A balanced eating habit will help to prevent nutrient deficiencies while on the Pill (see the Eating For Health chapter).

Things to watch out for while on the Pill

- Blood levels of vitamin A increase while on the Pill, so vitamin A supplements including cod liver oil, should never be taken with the Pill unless under practitioner supervision. The absorption of betacarotene (the precursor to vitamin A) from food, however, may be lower and so you should eat plenty of orange and yellow vegetables. If you want to get pregnant, or are pregnant, stop taking vitamin A as well as the Pill.

- If you are on the Pill or prescribed the Pill as well as

31

any other drug, discuss the possible effects with a doctor or at the local chemist.

- Some drugs can make the Pill a less powerful contraceptive, including some anti-epileptic drugs, some antibiotics and the anti-fungal medication, Griseofulvin. Some drugs are cleared more slowly from the body when women are on the Pill. Theophylline, the anti-asthma drug, is one of these.
- Painkillers with paracetamol, like Panadol, reduce the rate at which oestrogen is naturally cleared from the body and may lead to higher levels and more side effects from too much oestrogen.
- Women on thyroid hormones (such as Tertroxin) may need to increase their dose if they are also prescribed the Pill. Some sedatives, tranquillisers and antidepressant drugs may not work as well; others seem to have a stronger effect, such as the tricyclic anti-depressants Tofranil and Melipramine.

When to stop the Pill
Symptoms or conditions which indicate that the Pill should be stopped immediately include serious headaches, blood clots, or high blood pressure. You might consider stopping the Pill before going on a long plane flight too. Smoking while on the Pill increases the risk of developing those problems.

If you stop the Pill and don't start regular periods most doctors will not treat you unless you want to get pregnant. Then, a specialist gynaecologist might suggest fertility drugs like Clomid. (Side effects of this very strong drug should be discussed with your specialist.) Because of concerns about bone density when a woman is not menstruating, some doctors recommend that you go back on the Pill so that oestrogen levels are higher and bone health is maintained.

Progestogens

The commonly used progesterone-like drugs or 'progestogens' come from three classes—medroxyprogesterone acetate such as Provera, norethisterone such as Primulut N and dydrogesterone, or Duphaston. A separate class of drugs called Danazol will be discussed later in this section. Both Provera and Primulut N are used in the Pill, and are also prescribed for bleeding irregularities and for the menopause.

You may have heard of Depo Provera. This just means an injection of Provera—depo means injected—lasting three months. It is advertised by manufacturers as an easy, long-term contraception, but the drug can't be stopped early if side effects are a problem. There are other reliable tablet forms of contraception which have fewer side effects and can be stopped immediately a problem occurs, instead of having to wait three months until it wears off. One of the more serious side effects of long-term use of Depo Provera is bone loss, possibly leading to osteoporosis.

Another long-acting progestogen is called Implanon, an implant which is inserted into the fat of a non-dominant arm, and is active for three years. (Who knows where they put it if you're ambidextrous. Maybe they flip a coin.) Implanon has similar side effects to Depo Provera, but does not cause bone loss with long-term use. It can be removed if there are problems with common side effects such as bleeding, excess hair growth, or deepening of the voice. (Deepening of the voice caused by drugs is not always reversible.)

Progestogens are often prescribed for erratic heavy periods, even if the patient doesn't have irregularities in progesterone production. When you stop taking the drug, it causes complete shedding of the endometrium—it all comes out as a period—which often stops the abnormal bleeding. These drugs need to be given for about 21 days— usually from Day 5 to Day 25 of the menstrual cycle. (Day 1 is the first day of your period.) Progestogens are usually prescribed for between one and three menstrual cycles, but sometimes for longer. The androgen-like side effects and abnormal cholesterol levels associated with Primulut and the norethisterones restrict their use to no more than 6–12 months.

Provera and Duphaston (dydrogesterone) are the common progestogens used for endometriosis and can either be taken in the last part of the cycle, or taken continuously to create a pregnancy-like state with no period. About 30 per cent of women have spotting and breakthrough bleeding until the drug starts to work or the dose is adjusted. These drugs are relatively inexpensive (compared to some of the others used for endometriosis) and can give significant pain relief to some women without serious long-term side effects. Others can't tolerate the side effects at all.

Possible side effects
Progestogen side effects can include nausea, bloating, acne, breast tenderness, weight gain and mood changes

involving a lot of sudden, unexplained shouting (alright, maybe it was just me) which may be related to the blokey hormone effects of the drugs. The medroxyprogesterones such as Provera have fewer blokey hormone effects. Primulut and other norethisterones have mild oestrogenic, anabolic (growth promoting) and blokey hormone effects.

Provera and Duphaston can cause side effects in some women that are a real drag, or should we say drag queen, including increased hairiness, mood changes and a deeper voice. All the symptoms should go away after the drug use stops, except for the deepening of the voice. Singers and actors and people who want to sound like Betty Boop beware: use another drug if you can.

Fertility is not improved as a result of using progestogens. The return to a regular cycle may be delayed for many months.

What to take with progestogens

When side effects from progestogens are a problem, the B vitamins, magnesium, herbal diuretics or evening primrose oil, and essential fatty acids in the diet can sometimes reduce symptoms. For doses see the recommendations under the Pill, above. For information on magnesium, see page 145.

Danazol (danocrine)

Heavy stuff, Danazol needs to be carefully prescribed after careful consideration of the risks and benefits for each individual. For endometriosis, Danazol is prescribed in high doses (between 200 and 800 milligrams a day) to stop ovulation, suppress the period and cause the endometrium (both inside and out of the uterus) to shrink. Spotting can be a problem and is usually managed with a dose change.

On the helpful side, Danazol improves period pain and other pelvic pain and causes atrophy of endometriosis implants. It seems to have beneficial effects on the immune abnormalities, is better than other progestogens in improving fertility, and does not have an adverse effect on bone density. It has also been used to treat abnormally heavy bleeding, breast tenderness and cystic breast changes; and to improve lethargy, anxiety, and hunger frenzies associated with PMS. For these conditions, it is used at daily doses of around 200 milligrams which causes fewer side effects than higher doses and tends not to stop the period.

Possible side effects

Danazol is another progestogen which can cause pronounced blokey hormone effects such as male-pattern hair growth, deepening of the voice, weight gain, acne, and changes like smaller breasts, and an overgrown clitoris. These are reversible when drug use stops, except for a deeper voice, in some cases.

Severe and life-threatening strokes or thromboembolism (blood clots), and increased pressure inside the skull have also been reported with the use of Danazol; and long-term use may cause serious toxicity including jaundice and hepatitis. Some women find it also causes severe mood changes and symptoms like PMS. Some people take it with no trouble.

What to take with it

Side effects from Danazol are difficult to control, especially at the higher doses required for the treatment of endometriosis. However, trying the supplements suggested for the other progestogens can sometimes make the difference between being able to stay on the medication comfortably and feeling like you want to bite strangers in the street: 50–100 milligrams of vitamin B6 and 400–800 milligrams a day of magnesium seem to be particularly useful.

'Natural' progesterone

A popular medical alternative to the progestogens is progesterone, most commonly called 'natural progesterone' because its chemical make-up is identical to the progesterone made in the body.

This hormone preparation has been used for some time for PMS symptoms. Progesterone cannot be taken in a pill because it is very quickly broken down in the liver. So it has to be taken as either a vaginal pessary, a cream, an injection or a slow-release implant inserted under the skin. Progesterone has many enthusiastic supporters for its use in treating PMS and breast soreness even though controlled trials fail to show a better than placebo effect. It's used in the last week or two weeks before your period, depending on how severe the symptoms are.

It has also been recommended for endo, but compelling evidence that it may shrink endo implants is lacking.

GnRH agonists

These are the hormone-blocking drugs. We pause for a short message about how the body works. The hypothalamus gland in the brain releases a hormone called gonadotrophin-releasing hormone (GnRH). GnRH tells the pituitary gland to start pumping out important hormones which drive the menstrual cycle—luteinising hormone (LH) and follicle stimulating hormone (FSH).

Drugs with a similar chemical structure to GnRH are called GnRH analogues. GnRH analogues either mimic the action or stop you making your own GnRH. When taken continuously, a GnRH analogue stops ovulation and is then called a GnRH agonist—agonist means a competitor.

When taken for endometriosis, the drugs induce a temporary menopausal state. GnRH agonists are equally effective as Danazol in reducing the symptoms and the size of endometrial implants, and the side effects are said to be less severe.

Endometrial cysts usually return to their initial size four months after stopping drug treatment, making some sort of additional treatment necessary. GnRH agonists have no extra benefits in improving fertility.

GnRH agonists have also been trialled in combination with the Pill for premenstrual symptoms. These sorts of treatments are controversial because they're pretty heavy drugs, and are reserved for really feral cases of PMS. They are very occasionally used for abnormal bleeding which has failed to respond to other treatment.

GnRH agonists cannot be used as pills because of their chemical make-up. Instead, they are either given as an injection (Zoladex), usually once a month; or as a nostril spray (Synarel). They cause a menopausal state and stop periods during their use. Ovulation usually comes back within about a month of stopping the drugs.

Possible side effects of GnRH agonists
Menopausal symptoms such as hot flushes, dry vagina and headaches are common, and some women have difficulty with sex because of vaginal dryness and some women, come to mention it, find themselves less than interested in the whole idea of sex.

There is an early and significant bone density loss after starting on GnRH agonists. Radial bone density (measured in the wrist) is not affected, but the bone density of the spine shows significant changes. For some women, this may not be reversible and should be considered as part of their decision to use GnRH agonists. Oestrogen and progesterone given together might prevent bone density loss, but aggravate the condition that GnRH agonists were prescribed for.

Some people will develop ovarian cysts in the first two months of treatment with GnRH agonists, especially if they have a previous history of polycystic ovarian disease. These cysts will often disappear themselves as the treatment progresses, but can grow large enough to require surgery or going off the drug.

What to take with GnRH agonists
· Women who take GnRH agonists should ensure that their calcium and magnesium intake is high enough.

39

See info on calcium (page 148) and on magnesium (page 145).

- Plant oestrogens can help offset menopausal symptoms brought on by using the drugs (see info on plant (phyto) oestrogens, page 98).
- A water-based lubricant such as KY Jelly might make for more comfortable sex.
- Hot flushes are not so bad if you wear layers, such as a jacket or cardie you can throw off and on (somewhat in the style of a burlesque dancer, perhaps).
- Phyto-oestrogens can also help reduce the severity of hot flushes.

PAIN

Prostaglandins-inhibiting drugs like Ponstan are the most likely first suggestion for ordinary period pain, but also common are the Pill and some other types of painkillers. Sometimes, if the pain is severe and fails to respond to the usual treatments, very strong hormone drugs like Duphaston are used.

When period pain is really bad and all other treatments have been unsuccessful, the uterosacral nerve can be cut to destroy the perception of pain in the uterus. This is a drastic last step and is rarely used. If it is recommended to you, we hesitate to say run for the hills, but at the very least get a second opinion.

Which drug to choose depends on your medical history, the severity of your endo, which drugs you can tolerate easily and whether or not you want to get pregnant. The bottom line is that many prescribed drugs are strong and even toxic, to deal with the problem they target. The body can sometimes use a little help, either with something like a mineral, vitamin or herbal supplement from a natural therapist to offset side effects, or by finding another drug or brand of drug that you tolerate better. Always talk to your doctor if you are having a rough time: there are often alternatives.

Prostaglandins-inhibitors

These drugs inhibit the prostaglandins which cause the heavier periods and period pain from increased uterine muscle spasm. They can be bought without a prescription from a chemist. Aspirin is a well-known prostaglandins-inhibitor, but is not much chop for period pain. Some of the newer, more effective ones are Ponstan, Naprogesic, ACT 3 and Nurofen. Prostaglandins-inhibitors are absorbed quickly and can reduce pain in about half an hour. They can be used for the relief of period pain, including the moderate to severe period pain associated with endometriosis.

There seems to be no difference in effectiveness if the drugs are taken before the start of the period, but it's best to get on to them early if vomiting accompanies pain. Keep the dose in the lowest effective range. After you begin, take the drug strictly to recommended dosage— usually every six hours.

Women who have heavy periods and still ovulate regularly seem to respond better to these drugs than women who are not ovulating. The drugs also seem to work better in combination with the Pill or progesterone tablets, and some doctors recommend these treatments be combined.

41

These drugs are also occasionally recommended for PMS, but you shouldn't take them for longer than seven days at a time, so they're no good for the many women who experience PMS for more than a week before their period.

Prostaglandins-inhibitors do not actually reverse the prostaglandins imbalance which causes heavy periods, pain or PMS and will have to be used indefinitely until the cause(s) of the imbalance are found and dealt with, because the drug just attacks the symptom, not the cause.

Prostaglandins-inhibitors only control symptoms while they're around. This is not a very alluring prospect, especially since there are many side effects.

Possible side effects of prostaglandins-inhibitors
About a quarter of people using prostaglandins-inhibitors have problems with the gastro-intestinal system. Symptoms can include nausea, vomiting, stomach pain, indigestion, diarrhoea, heartburn, abdominal cramps, constipation, abdominal bloating and wind. These drugs should always be taken with food to try to minimise the risk of gastric ulceration. Steer clear of them if you have a history of gastro-intestinal disease. A number of other complaints can be aggravated by the use of prostaglandins-inhibitors and they may cause problems if you have poor liver function, asthma, clotting disorders, lupus, and heart disease. Prostaglandins-inhibitors can mask the signs of infection and should not be taken when period pain is known or suspected to be caused by pelvic inflammatory disease.

What to take with prostaglandins-inhibitors
Slippery elm can help to prevent gastric ulceration associated with these drugs. One teaspoon mixed into apple juice, or into equal quantities of apple juice mixed with yoghurt, and taken at the same time as the drug, helps to protect the stomach lining.

Other pain medications
Many women 'self-medicate' with painkillers ranging from aspirin and paracetamol, through to codeine and other preparations. These are rarely recommended or prescribed by doctors for period pain any more for good reason—they don't even begin to strike at the reasons for the symptoms, or the specific pain you're experiencing. Repeated overuse of painkillers is associated with kidney damage and other health problems. It is always best to have your problem diagnosed and then speak to a specialist or a family doctor about the most appropriate, effective painkiller.

FERTILITY

Not everyone wants to have children. Some are ambivalent; some want it desperately. This is for those who are interested.

Fertility problems must be treated by a fertility expert. Natural therapies and medical treatments can be used in tandem but each practitioner needs to know what the other is doing. And it is important to get a diagnosis before treatment. Any medical treatment works best in conjunction with other help such as counselling, natural therapies and self care strategies such as a healthier lifestyle and specific diet changes. GPs can advise you on beginning to try to get pregnant, but if you know you've had endo, or have been trying for some months without success, get a referral to a fertility specialist. The older you are, the earlier you should come for help, especially after you reach 35.

As is the case with natural therapies, surgical and drug treatment of endo will not necessarily increase fertility: it very much depends on each individual. Some women do have conditions which are preventing conception, particularly severe damage from endo, that can be quickly corrected with surgery. But as with any treatment there is no guarantee, only educated guesses.

Pinpointing ovulation

A doctor, or natural therapist trained in this area, should help you to identify your most fertile times each month so that you can maximise your chances of conceiving. Methods used range from simply guessing which days you'll be most fertile, to tracking mucus in the vagina around the time of ovulation and keeping temperature charts. These are called basal body temperature charts—this means your temperature is taken first thing in the morning before you move around or get out of bed. An old-fashioned mercury thermometer rather than a digital one works best, stuck under your tongue. A chart of your temperature marked on a graph showing the days of your period, and a sample of the

 44

mucus can be used by your health practitioner for more specific advice.

If this is not successful within a few months (if you're approaching 40) or, say, six months if you're a lot younger, it will need looking into. Get a referral from your GP to a fertility expert.

Diagnosis of infertility

There's not much point treating infertility unless the problem is diagnosed. If you have endometriosis, and problems with fertility, likely causes include adhesions that are blocking your Fallopian tubes or inflammatory processes which seem to be able to prevent conception. (The problem may even lie with the bloke involved, not you.) Other causes include an underlying problem such as polycystic ovarian syndrome, or pelvic inflammatory disease; being underweight or overweight, or a problem with the sperm. Many people diagnosed as infertile surprise themselves and everyone else when they exhaust their treatment options, give up and suddenly have a baby through natural means. Others spend years of heartache and grief and must adjust to other ways of being important in the lives of children.

Those who have been diagnosed with an infertility problem should see a specialist fertility counsellor—these people deal with the emotional and the physical possibilities open to you, and are well connected with any medical advances and other useful information. Most women's hospitals have a fertility counsellor who can help you identify your symptoms and problem and recommend treatment. See the What Now? chapter for books on maximising your chance to conceive as well as other counselling and medical help.

Surgery

Doctors may opt for a laparoscopy to ensure there is nothing blocking the Fallopian tubes, and no other identifiable physical reason for infertility that can be identified and perhaps mended.

Clomid and other fertility drugs

Doctors sometimes prescribe a fairly hefty fertility drug called Clomid which can result in the ovaries producing many eggs. Side effects from fertility drugs include mood changes, nausea, headaches, and occasionally abdominal pain, especially when the ovary has been overstimulated, called ovarian hyperstimulation. Other drugs that mimic the action of the central, controlling hormones produced in the hypothalamus and pituitary gland in the brain can also cause the ovary to produce several follicles (eggs). These can be collected and fertilised in a test tube (see IVF below) or the woman might see if she can get one of the eggs fertilised in the time honoured way in the privacy of her own home.

IVF

The *in vitro* fertilisation technique (meaning using glass, in this case a test tube) is used to help women conceive outside of their uterus. In a laboratory, sperm is introduced to an egg which has been taken from a woman's ovary. The fertilised egg, or eggs, are then implanted into the woman's uterus. It may take many tries before a successful pregnancy is achieved, or it may not be successful. Which women may have this treatment, and how many tries they can have, is usually determined by state government legislation. IVF treatment can be painful, both physically and emotionally. It is often suggested for women with serious blockage(s) or damage to the Fallopian tubes which makes it impossible for sperm to get to the eggs in normal circumstances. Bypassing the blockage by fertilising the eggs in a test tube and then placing the embryo in the uterus is sometimes the best or only option open to women with severe endometriosis. To maximise the chances of a viable pregnancy the IVF doctor will often implant two embryos. This can mean that important decisions must be made with regard to the realities of a multiple birth or selective terminations.

DEPRESSION AND MOOD SWINGS

Anti-depressants and anxiolytics

A variety of anti-depressants and anxiolytics (anti-anxiety drugs) are sometimes used for mood disorders associated with period problems, particularly PMS, endometriosis and meno-pause. As a general rule it's best to stay right away from them as a treatment for PMS-induced

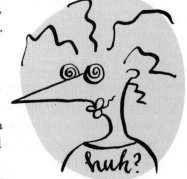

mood swings. They treat only the symptoms of depression if they treat anything at all and not the underlying hormonal cause. As you can tell by the general tone of this book, we'd much rather you got to the cause of your problem instead of just tinkering with the symptoms. It might sound a bit jolly hockey sticks, but studies have shown that a good, brisk walk for 30 minutes can improve moods as much as some drugs, so why not try that first?

Sometimes with endo the depression can get more entrenched and anti-depressant drugs may be necessary. These include Zoloft, Effexor and Cipramil, but there are many others. Alternatives include the nervine herbs such as St John's Wort in precise doses (see the Natural Therapy chapter), and counselling. A good counsellor may help you unravel the frustrations and disappointments often associated with endometriosis that can lead to feeling worthless, depressed and anxious. The minor tranquillisers, such as the benzodiazepines (Valium) can simply add to the fatigue and lethargy often associated with hormonal changes. If you have problems with depression or anxiety that are severe and unrelenting you may be better off if you see a psychiatrist who will monitor your moods and your drugs.

ADHESIONS

Doctors are now very aware of the problem of adhesions—surgery is used to remove the adhesions caused by endometriosis cysts and deposits inside the pelvis. Specialist surgeons take care to try to prevent new adhesions by

 48

the healing and fusing of areas after their own surgery. This is done by using products such as Interceed, a tiny sheet that can be placed between healing organs and that melts away of its own accord when the organs have healed up without fusing together. Adhesions can't always be prevented, but vitamin E can be helpful (see the Natural Therapy Solutions chapter on page 64.)

SURGERY FOR DIAGNOSIS AND TREATMENT

'Minor' surgery is the only known foolproof way of finding out for sure if you have endo, and of delivering effective treatment. Major surgery can be the only way of treating some very severe cases. So, if you've gotta, you've gotta, but don't be afraid of getting a second opinion, or more if you like, before you agree. Except in emergency situations, surgery should be seen as a last resort. In this section we explain the most common procedures.

Whatever surgery you're having, make sure you read the hints below about preparing for surgery and better recovery. These days you can be shovelled in and out of hospital so fast, you'll need all the help you can get in recovering. (Don't feel you have to go home the same day, and if you do, make sure somebody can care for you properly. If you're going home alone or to a houseful of screaming kids who need looking after—don't be bullied and insist on the extra day in hospital. The after-effects of general anaesthetic are not to be sneezed at.)

Good pre-operative strategies can make all the difference to recovering quickly and easily from even a major operation. And remember, even the most hot-shot surgeon or anaesthetist who answers all your questions could be very pressed for time, or have a shocking manner, and find it difficult to explain things in ways that make sense to you, or to be a warm presence at a scary time.

Are you making the right decision? What are your future options? It can really help to be in touch with other people who have been through this, or even to read their accounts of their operations and experiences—time to hit the support groups, in person, or on the internet (see the What Now? chapter)!

When should I have surgery?

The most common recommendation is for a laparoscopy to confirm a tentative diagnosis of endometriosis. Laparoscopies are often also used for an inspection to see if there's an obvious reason for fertility problems.

If the patient has given prior permission, any endometrial lesions and cysts that are found can be be removed then, so you don't have to undergo surgery twice. (There's not much worse than waking up after an operation and being told, 'Yes, there's something in there that should come out, so as soon as you've recovered from this op, let's just go in again!' as once happened to the flightier author of this book, who changed to another doctor at the speed of light.)

Endo cysts and patches can be destroyed by the surgeon using different methods: burned away with diathermy electrical current; vaporised by lasers and/or cut out with a scalpel. The surgeon will be intent on 'getting it all' during the operation. A combined method using both the cutting away and the laser usually provides pain relief for patients.

Occasionally, some women will need detailed, microscopic surgery to remove adhesions from organs such as the Fallopian tubes. Really serious endo that has damaged internal organs or endo causing pain that refuses to respond to any treatment may require a hysterectomy. This is obviously not a decision to be taken lightly and should be considered only as a last resort.

Anaesthetics

If you're having general anaesthetic you will need to stay in hospital for a minimum of four hours and maybe longer, depending on what procedures you undergo. Anaesthetics are evolving all the time, and have been since they used whisky or a swift blow to the noggin. 'General' anaesthetics will render you unconscious for the duration of the surgery. Different 'generals' are used—anaesthetists often have their own favourites. Some people react badly to anaesthetics—if you have a second operation after a bad experience recovering from anaesthetic, find out what you had last time and tell the anaesthetist to try something different. It's increasingly popular to skip the 'pre-med' relaxing shot of pethidine or other drugs, such as Scopolomine, used to dry up secretions. It's now believed that people recover more quickly from anaesthetic after an operation if they don't have a pre-med. Never lie to your anaesthetist about how much you weigh, how much alcohol you drink or how many cigarettes you smoke. This will affect the amount of anaesthetic and drugs you need during surgery.

Laparoscopy

A look around the pelvic organs, usually searching for problems like blocked Fallopian tubes, endometriosis or cysts of some kind. Many kinds of treatment may be performed at the same time, such as removal of cysts, and laser destruction of endometriosis implants.

Anaesthetic

General, in hospital.

Procedure

The surgeon makes two or more small incisions to insert the look-around instrument, called a laparoscope. This thin, pencil-like instrument has fibre-optics through which the operator can view the inner organs. There is usually one incision under the navel and another just above the pubic bone. The abdomen is usually filled with a gas so that it is pumped up with an 'air' making it easier for the surgeon to see each individual organ, and there's more room to move the laparoscope around. At the end of the procedure, most of the gas is forced out, but some stays in the abdominal cavity and can cause pain or discomfort until it eventually dissipates, which can be after a few days. The pressure of the gas affects nerves, and can cause 'referred' pain in the shoulders.

Minor surgical procedures can be performed during a laparoscopy, such as removing patches of endometriosis with laser (which vaporises) or diathermy (burning off with electrical current), the removal of small ovarian cysts, and the removal of adhesions. These procedures usually involve only a day in hospital; and pain and post-operative complications are minimal because the incisions are small. But it is *not* trivial. It's surgery.

Duration

Sometimes you can go home the same day, sometimes the next day, depending on what had to be done. A quick look around is one thing, but additional surgery like laser treatment will add on to your recovery time. Recovery time is usually several days depending on the extent of the additional surgery and the type of complaint treated. Even though the external wounds can be quite small, the internal organs might take a while to recover. Pain is a good indicator of how much to do and when rest is needed. Listen to your body. See the advice below on pre- and post-op care: it's important.

Laparotomy

It's generally accepted by specialist endometriosis surgeons that a laparotomy—an abdominal operation with a much bigger incision and recovery time—is outdated as a method for getting at most cases of endo. Sometimes, though, if a large cyst has to be removed, and the damage or adhesions is very extensive, a laparoscopy does not give the surgeon enough room to manoeuvre, and a laparotomy is performed. The recovery time will be longer if the incision and surgery is more extensive than expected.

Hysterectomy

This procedure, the removal of the uterus, is a last resort for unresponsive endometriosis, for obvious reasons. If you don't have a uterus, you can't make endometrium. It's always wise to get at least one more opinion before proceeding. Firstly it means you will not be able to have children afterwards. Even if this is not an issue, it is major surgery with many physical and psychological implications, which should be discussed with your doctor.

Removal of the ovaries as well as the uterus is often recommended. Removing the ovaries can prevent or slow down the growth of the oestrogen-responsive endometriosis but, of course, means you will become menopausal. According to medical wisdom, a hysterectomy which takes the uterus and leaves the ovaries shouldn't cause any interruption in ovarian activity—but up to a third of women who have this surgery do have menopausal symptoms. If menopause isn't brought on immediately by a hysterectomy, on average, it will come on five years earlier than in women who still have their uterus.

Anaesthetic
General, in hospital.

Procedure
A hysterectomy is the removal of the uterus, but the removal of the uterus and Fallopian tubes and ovaries is generally also known as a hysterectomy. A 'total hysterectomy' usually means that the cervix is taken as well as the uterus, and a 'sub-total' hysterectomy usually means the cervix is left alone. Sometimes doctors talk about a 'partial

hysterectomy' (removal of the uterus but not the ovaries). In the past, it was more common to have a hysterectomy operation in which the ovaries and uterus were both surgically removed. (If you let them, surgeons will refer to this as a bilateral salpingo-oophorectomy.)

Make sure you understand exactly what your doctor means when the word hysterectomy is used. The operation can be done by making an incision in the abdomen and cutting out the uterus; or by entering the body through the vagina with surgical instruments, cutting away the uterus, and pulling it out through the vagina. (Sorry to get a bit graphic, but that's what happens.) A hysterectomy for endometriosis will probably be done through an abdominal incision if there are multiple adhesions which make vaginal removal too difficult.

Duration

This is a major operation. It usually takes three-quarters of an hour to an hour, but can take several hours depending on possible complications. The amount of pain you'll experience will be partially related to the size of the wound, but recovery time is also determined by how fit and healthy you are and how easily you can move around after surgery. You will probably be in hospital for between five and ten days. Colicky bowel pain can be very severe after a hysterectomy and many women say this is the worst part of the whole experience; see the hints under Preparing for Surgery to get tips on how to alleviate this problem.

Preparing for surgery

The following pre-surgery hints will help you to improve wound healing and reduce wound infections; assist with getting up and around again as quickly as possible; and cut down on the common discomfort of bowel problems after surgery, caused by your inside bits being disturbed. The hints will help in any abdominal surgery, including hysterectomy, myomectomy, laparoscopy, laser surgery, laparotomy or caesarean section. Check them with your surgeon.

- Give up smoking—for good if you can, but at least for two weeks before the operation. This will reduce your risk of post-operative chest infections.
- A few dietary changes in the week before surgery can help to prevent or reduce the symptoms of bowel problems afterwards.
- The seed breakfast (see page 102) should be started about one week before the operation and continued as soon as solid foods can be eaten after surgery.
- Eat daily salads of grated raw carrot and beetroot or a medium-sized cooked beetroot.
- Yoghurt or cultured milk drinks colonise the bowel with healthy bacteria and cut down on painful wind. Drink or eat about one cup a day of yoghurt with live cultures and no sugar. (Jalna, Hakea and Gippsland are good brands with low-fat options.)
- Avoid refined sugars which tend to increase bowel fermentation and wind.

- Avoid foods which usually cause you wind or constipation or diarrhoea.
- If you already have irritable bowel syndrome or suffer from sensitive bowels: in the week before the op, have three to six cups daily of a special herbal tea combination. Make up a jar with equal parts of *Melissa officinalis* (lemon balm), *Matricaria recutita* (chamomile) and *Mentha piperita* (peppermint tea). Use 2 teaspoons of the mixture for each cup of tea. Take it with you to hospital, and continue taking it for the week after the operation. Stay off normal tea and coffee while you're recuperating.
- Post-operative nausea is relieved by common ginger root. The usual dose is between ½ and 1 gram every four hours, in tablet form, or between 10 and 20 drops as an oral fluid extract. Organise to take this to the hospital with you to start using as soon as you can after the surgery, but check with the medical staff first.
- Get your muscles going. Poor muscle strength and agility can slow down recovery because getting out of bed and walking around is much more difficult. Weak leg and abdominal muscles can be improved by specific exercises such as yoga exercises, squats, walking, sit-ups and gym work. About a month is usually needed to dramatically improve muscle strength but even a few days before the op is better than nothing.
- Vitamin C has been shown to improve wound healing time. Start at least one week before surgery on about 2 grams a day and keep going for three to four weeks afterwards.

- Make sure you're getting enough zinc. A lot of women don't. Zinc supplements also have a beneficial effect on wound healing, but probably only in zinc-deficient people. Start a good zinc supplement, such as around 75–150 milligrams of zinc chelate a day with food for two or three weeks before the operation and continue for about two weeks afterwards.
- Vitamin E, which prevents internal scar tissue formation (adhesions), is useful when fertility must be conserved following surgery. Doses of around 100–250 IU should be taken two weeks before the surgery but stopped two days before the operation. This is a relatively small dose, because of a very slight risk of increased bleeding during surgery. Once you can eat again after the operation you can take doses of around 400 or 500 IU a day until you're recovered. This will reduce the risk of post-operative blood clots. Vitamin E cream can also be rubbed into the wound to speed up healing and reduce scarring.

Recovering from surgery

People have forgotten how to convalesce. With the increase in laser surgery, and the resulting shorter hospital stays, some patients are sent home the day after surgery or even the day of the operation.

Many women start housework, child care or go back to work within days of surgical procedures and then wonder why they spend the rest of the year feeling so awful. The financial strains on the average household also mean that many people feel they 'can't afford' to convalesce properly.

Don't take too much notice of standard doctors' predictions of 'you'll be back at the gym in a week' or 'you'll be up and walking by tomorrow'. Everybody is different. Our completely unscientific, informal survey of women who have had abdominal surgery revealed that all of them took longer to recover than their doctors suggested they would, and so they felt there was something wrong with their constitution, not with what the doctor told them.

Any surgery can take longer than expected, with much intrusive moving around of your inside bits. The standard recovery prediction then becomes even less relevant to you, but sometimes you won't be given a re-assessment of your convalescent time.

Recovery times vary considerably between individuals and are influenced by factors such as smoking, lack of previous fitness, an inability to take it easy and let the body heal, having to get up and look after the kids or go back to work before you're ready, as well as more surgery than was originally planned.

It's better to be guided by pain and stamina and to do a little more every day than to resume former levels of work and exercise too quickly. In other words—go by how you feel, not by a standard information sheet given out by the hospital, which may be based on estimates or best-case scenarios.

When the body is under stress or recovering from an illness, it needs heaps more nutrients than usual. Unfortunately, this often happens just when you've lost your appetite. (Any stress, whether it be from surgery, difficult times, a car accident, or too much work, has a similar effect on the body's need for nutrients.)

Being physically active after the procedure improves recovery time and stamina, and reduces the risk of blood clots and respiratory infections. This does not mean you can start doing aerobics the day after. It means you start shuffling around in your slippers as soon as you can and build up from there.

- Your recovering body needs a boost of protein, the B vitamins—particularly vitamin B5 (pantothenic acid)—vitamin C, potassium, magnesium and zinc. You can have a daily vitamin B complex tablet which has 50 milligrams of B5 and B6, with a multi-mineral supplement and 1–2 grams of powdered vitamin C until you feel on top of things again.
- To keep energy steady, eat small but frequent meals of complex carbohydrate (potato, rice, bread, oatmeal and pasta), combined with small amounts of protein such as yoghurt, cheese, tofu, hommos, tuna or egg until your normal appetite and bowel function comes back.
- Avoid any food which acts as a 'body stressor', such as caffeine, refined sugars and huge strawberry daiquiris, until you've recovered.
- Some exercise is vital. Exercise every second day allows for one day of recovery after energy expenditure. As strength improves, exercise every day will increase stamina and a sense of wellbeing. Exercise should be taken at a much slower pace. People tend to overestimate their capabilities so a good rule of thumb is to start at half the level you imagine you could comfortably manage now; if it is too little, no harm will be

done. Long slow distance exercise is best—especially walking.

- Simple, easily digested soups and 'energy drinks' provide concentrated nutrients.
- Have one serve of a cooked green leafy vegetable such as spinach, Chinese cabbage or silverbeet every day during the recovery period.
- Never skip breakfast and have a cooked breakfast (porridge, egg on toast, cooked rice cereal, vegetable soup) at least every second day.
- Use the 'suggested menus' given for the hypoglycaemia diet (see page 93).

Soups are useful recovery foods. The best types are ones based on grains, especially barley and rice; legumes, such as tofu, orange lentils, fresh soya beans and red kidney beans (but not if they give you wind); or root vegies like potato, carrot and sweet potato.

Chicken broth
Yes, the old standby, traditional comfort food. Use free-range chicken carcasses if you can. The broth can be prepared with a particular flavour; for example, Thai (lemongrass, lime leaves, galangal and chilli), or Western (celery, bay leaves, onion, carrot and peppercorns).

High-protein drinks
High-protein drinks are useful meal substitutes or for between meals, particularly if you don't feel hungry and you're having trouble digesting:

ALMOND SMOOTHIE

2 dessertspoons almond meal
1 teaspoon rice bran
1 teaspoon wheatgerm

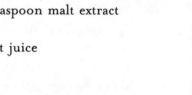

Blend with:
1 cup commercial soya milk (Bonsoy,
    Aussie Soy, Vitasoy) and 1 teaspoon malt extract
or
½ cup yoghurt and ½ cup fruit juice

BERRY DRINK

½ punnet blueberries, strawberries, raspberries or other
    berry fruit in season
½ to ¾ cup yoghurt or soya milk (yoghurt and berries
    tend to be fairly tangy and may not be to everyone's
    liking)
1 dessertspoon almond meal, ground cashews, or seeds
    (the 'seed mix' for irritable bowel syndrome is suit-
    able; see page 102)

Blend together until smooth.

TOFU DRINKS

50 grams soft tofu

Blend with any of the following combinations:

6 dried apricots (soaked overnight in a cup of water) and
    the water they have been soaked in
2 dessertspoons almond meal
1 teaspoon slippery elm powder

or

1 banana

1 teaspoon slippery elm powder *or* 1 teaspoon rice bran

1 dessertspoon almond meal

1 cup fruit juice

or

1 glass freshly squeezed orange juice

1–2 dessertspoons almond meal *or* ground cashew nuts
    or 'seed mix'

1 teaspoon slippery elm powder

Natural Therapy Solutions

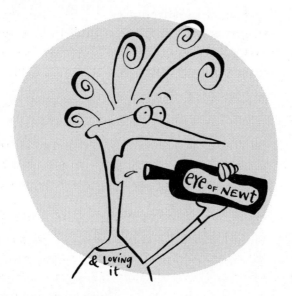

The natural therapist's treatment of endo aims (not necessarily in this order) to:

- decrease pain and regulate your prostaglandins;
- regulate hormones by treating PMS and bringing down relatively high levels of oestrogen;
- help with depression and mood swings;
- reduce formation of adhesions;
- treat immune system irregularities;
- improve fertility, if that is an aim.

64

The big factors here in deciding on treatment are the amount of pain you have and whether you want to get pregnant. And if the pain is really severe, then knocking that on the head has to be the first priority. We recommend a combined approach with a specialist gynaecologist as well as a natural therapist. Make sure everyone in your health team knows that this is what you're doing. You might have surgery and follow up with herbs, or surgery then six months of drugs and then herbs or dietary changes. Remember endo often recurs and natural therapies are good to help prevent this. Let's have a look at the main principles in detail, but first, we get stern for a paragraph:

If your herbalist is not experienced, they should consult Ruth's text book, *Women, Hormones and the Menstrual Cycle*, for students and practitioners, which contains recommended doses and usages of the relevant herbs. Alternatively, get in touch with endo self-help groups (there's a list at the back of the book), who may be able to help you contact a natural therapist with a specialty in endometriosis. Do not self-prescribe. Many doses and combinations are finely calibrated and can have opposite, or no effect at all, if misused. Despite some people's temptation to regard them all as benign, 'natural' compounds, the misuse of herbs can be just as dangerous as any misuse of drugs. Many of them must not be used if there is a chance you may be pregnant, for example. Treatment options you can prescribe on your own (take two hot-water bottles and call yourself in the morning) are in the Self Care chapter.

PAIN

Herbs

Everyone experiences period pain differently and has their own combination of symptoms. Herbal formulas which are individually prescribed should try to deal with as many of these symptoms as possible. Over-the-counter herbal remedies for period pain can't have exactly the right combination of herbs for everyone.

In herbal medicine, the emphasis comes off painkillers and onto underlying reasons for the pain. All of the herbal and other remedies treat the cause of the pain—the prostaglandins imbalance, the uterine muscle spasm, the hormone imbalance and the inflammatory responses. Fish oils reduce period pain caused by prostaglandins and leukotriene imbalance. In some cases of endo, much of the pain is from the bowel (more of which later). It can be quite complicated to design a remedy for period pain. You'll need a specialist herbalist to prescribe your individual formula. You're likely to be prescribed a 'cocktail' of the following herbs, tailored to your individual diagnosis.

- The uterine tonics are possibly the most important group of herbs for the pain of endo. They are given to improve 'uterine tone', which is the ability of the uterus to maintain orderly and regular activity. Uterine tone is mainly regulated by the prostaglandins, and the prostaglandins are largely kept in check by hormone levels, so uterine tonics are prescribed in combination with hormone-regulating herbs for best effects. Because the uterine tonics help maintain normal activity of the uterine muscle, they are responsible for making period pain easier. *Angelica sinensis* (Dang Gui) is the principal herb used for endometriosis; *Caulophyllum thalictroides* (blue cohosh), and *Rubus idaeus* (raspberry leaves) are good, too. *Chamaelirium luteum* (helonias), once the favoured uterine tonic for endo is endangered and *Angelica sinensis* is now usually used as a substitute.

- The anti-spasmodic herbs include *Viburnum opulus* (cramp bark) and *V. prunifolium* (black haw), *Caulophyllum thalictroides* (blue cohosh), *Dioscorea villosa* (wild yam), and *Paeonia lactiflora* (white peony). These herbs reduce uterine muscle spasm and relieve pain. Some combinations work better than others. *Paeonia lactiflora* is usually combined with *Glycyrrhiza glabra* (liquorice) to obtain the best effect. *Caulophyllum thalictroides* is best with *Viburnum opulus* when the spasm seems to be localised to the cervix, resulting in acute crampy flow with very little flow. There are many other examples of herbal combinations and this is not an area for the untrained. All the herbs here should only be prescribed by a specialist herbalist. As Auntie Myrtle always said, never let an amateur near your uterus, dear.

- Emmenagogues have an expulsive effect on the uterus, and can speed up or 'bring on' the period flow. They are indicated for congestive symptoms which include heavy dragging pain, especially when the period is late. They should always be prescribed with uterine tonics—and without really wanting to bore you—we have to say again, by a qualified herbalist.

- Warming herbs: two are especially specific for the pelvic region: *Zingiber officinale* (ginger) and *Cinnamomum zeylanicum* (cinnamon). Both can be added to a herbal mix in the form of a tincture, or taken as a tea, either alone, with other therapeutic herbs or in an ordinary cuppa.

- Nervine (relaxing) herbs are useful to help the action of the anti-spasmodic and pain-killing herbs, and also if anxiety or tension accompany the pain. Some nervine herbs are also anti-spasmodics, the best being *Valeriana officinalis*, *Piscidia erythrina*, *Corydalis ambigua*, *Verbena officinalis* and *Matricaria recutita* (chamomile).

- Anodyne, or pain-reducing herbs. *Corydalis ambigua* from the Chinese Materia Medica is the most potent of these, and can be used for pain anywhere in the body. It also reduces heavy period flow. Other important anodynes for period pain are *Piscidia erythrina*, *Lactuca virosa* and *Anemone pulsatilla*.

- Prostaglandins-inhibiting herbs include *Zingiber officinale* (ginger), *Tanacetum parthenium* (feverfew) and *Curcuma longa*. There are probably others, but there is little research in this area.

- Herbs which regulate the hormone levels. The most valuable of the herbal hormone regulators is *Vitex agnus castus*, which is very useful for endometriosis and congestive period pain, especially if PMS is also a problem. Vitex is a very difficult herb to prescribe successfully and should be prescribed by a specialist practitioner.

- Other herbs include *Paeonia lactiflora* and *P. suffruticosa* and *Cimicifuga racemosa* which are anti-spasmodics and may also competitively inhibit the activity of oestrogen; and *Verbena officinalis* which is a sedative and has been traditionally used for hormonal period disorders.
- Congestive period pain, the heavy, dull, dragging type of pain experienced by many women before their period, is often improved by taking liver herbs or bitters such as *Berberis vulgaris* which is also an emmenagogue. Other liver herbs include *Taraxacum officinale* (dandelion), *Silybum marianum* (St Mary's thistle).
- Herbs for spasmodic or congestive period pain accompanied by constipation and irritable bowel syndrome. The 'aperient' (laxative) herbs such as *Cassia senna* (senna pods), *Rhamnus purshiana* (cascara) and *Aloe barbadensis* (aloe) can be used but will often aggravate spasm in the uterus if taken during the period. Beware of laxatives bought from the chemist with these elements, as the effects can be rather, ahem, violent.

By far the best method to treat constipation is to increase the level of fibre and fluids in the diet. (A sensible high-fibre diet is included in the Eating for Health chapter.) Irritable bowel syndrome often becomes worse around the period and can aggravate period pain—sometimes it is even mistaken for period pain. (See the irritable bowel syndrome diet on page 102.)

Acupuncture

Acupuncture can help some period pain. It involves the insertion of needles into the skin which sounds scary, but if you breathe in really quickly as each needle goes in you don't feel a thing. Obviously what you'll need is an experienced acupuncturist, not some mad pal with an old school compass—the placing of the needles is very precise. The treatments are usually given twice a week.

Chiropractic and osteopathy

Some chiropractors and osteopaths believe that period pain can be aggravated by pressure on the spinal nerves that supply the uterus. They treat this problem by manipulating the lower back. Any likely positive response should be obvious within one or two treatments.

Massage

Massage can relieve or aggravate period pain. A masseur specialising in this area is essential. Make sure you understand the difference between therapeutic massage, a relaxing massage, or any other massage claimed to have 'healing' effects.

Regulating the prostaglandins

The body uses Omega-3 fatty acids to balance leukotrienes and thromboxanes, and Omega-6 fatty acids to balance prostaglandins. The essential fatty acids found in oily fish have the greatest impact on period pain and retrograde flow caused by prostaglandins or leukotriene imbalance.

For the best healthy effects, you need to eat more essential fatty acids and less of the 'bad oils' which interfere with them. See Bad Fats and Good Fats on page 118.

The herbs *Tanacetum parthenium* (feverfew) and *Zingiber officinale* (ginger) also have prostaglandins-inhibiting effects and can improve period pain. According to herbal traditions, feverfew is classed as a Cold herb, ginger is Hot. As most period pain is made worse by cold, feverfew is often combined with ginger. Again, these must be prescribed by a specialist herbal practitioner.

More about what prostaglandins do and how they work if you're interested, otherwise skip it

To work properly, ovulation, periods and childbirth all depend on the hormones to behave themselves. It is not so well known that they also rely on some complicated, hormone-like substances called prostaglandins to behave themselves as well. It may help to think of prostaglandins as a large family of hormone-like substances which perform many functions throughout the body.

Prostaglandins are made by the body to control heaps of different functions, for example, bleeding, clotting, anti-inflammatory action and muscle spasms. This makes them big players in the menstrual cycle, what with all that experience in stopping and starting bleeding and controlling crampy things.

Some prostaglandins might become too dominant in cases of infection, inflammation, allergy, hormone variations or poor diet. These imbalances may be temporary, or continue indefinitely, and are believed to be causes of period pain, heavy periods, PMS and endometriosis.

The prostaglandin family is really a sub-group of an extended family of microscopic substances found in most tissues called the eicosanoids (I-ko-san-oids). In the eicosanoid extended family, there are two clans—the large and well-known family called the prostaglandins, and a smaller branch of rellies called the leukotrienes.

The prostaglandin family is itself made up of even smaller families, like nuclear families in an extended clan. These families include the prostacyclins and the thromboxanes as well as a group of individual prostaglandins. Each of the members of the extended family has a broad role to play: as we've said, the prostaglandins influence blood clotting, the activity of muscles and the inflammatory responses throughout the body; on the other hand the thromboxanes are involved with blood clotting and blood vessel activity; and the leukotrienes are regulators of inflammatory and allergic reactions. Whenever you bleed, get a scab, throw up or have a muscle spasm, there's a prostaglandin leukotriene or thromboxane working overtime.

Within each of the thromboxane, prostaglandins and leukotriene families, each of the members has its own more detailed role. As with all families, some of the members tend to be nuisances, others are more useful. Just as some rellies are liable to go off the deep end at any given time (especially Christmas), some of the rellies in the prostaglandin family can go a bit feral from time to time. And then there are the distant rellies—some of whom can be unreliable. For example, one of the leukotrienes will start some of the processes of inflammation, and another one, either a close or distant clan relative, will have the role of calming everything down.

The prostaglandins do various conflicting jobs in the menstrual cycle, so they need to be in balance. One type of prostaglandin stops platelets from clumping together and dilates blood vessels, which causes heavier period bleeding. Another prostaglandin strongly increases muscle contraction, but in the Fallopian tube, it causes relaxation. Another one is always complaining that the young people of today get it too good. Sorry, that's one of my relatives.

Rogue prostaglandins can be responsible for the crampy type of period pain, because some prostaglandins cause blood vessels in the endometrium to constrict, as well as causing muscle spasm. When these are too dominant, they can cause period pain from the cramping muscle.

And in general, leukotrienes stimulate uterus contractions, so when some of these leukotrienes go into overdrive, the contractions also cause crampy period pain. One type of leukotriene attracts white cells to inflamed tissues and is found in high levels when women have endometriosis.

Balancing prostaglandins

- Essential fatty acid supplements, such as evening primrose oil or star flower oil. Doses of 3 grams of evening primrose oil containing 216 milligrams of linoleic acid and 27 milligrams of gamma linoleic acid (GLA) or the equivalent taken daily from mid-cycle until the period may be useful in regulating prostaglandins. You'll need vitamin B6 and zinc to make it work. Diet

73

can also be altered to take in more essential fatty acids (see page 120).

- Vitamin E: between 100 and 600 International Units (IU) daily can also help balance prostaglandins.
- Eat more often—a 'grazing' or hypoglycaemic diet. Little meals more often is the go. The positive effects may be related to stabilisation of blood sugars as well as to indirect influences on progesterone. (See the hypoglycaemia diet on page 92.)
- Many of the symptoms of PMS have been attributed to magnesium deficiency (there's a magnesium info page in the Eating for Health chapter, page 145). If that sounds like you, eat more magnesium-containing foods and restrict dairy products.

PMS

To try to break it down a bit, PMS has been divided into five sub-groups by a research doctor, each based on a different hormonal, biochemical and/or nutritional cause. Treatments for PMS are based on the five different sub-groups and are composed of a mixture of supplements and dietary advice, herbal remedies and lifestyle changes. Do not self-prescribe the herbs listed below. The type of PMS you have is often an indication of what kind of

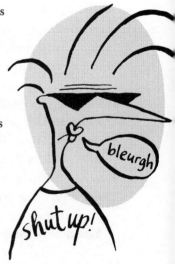

hormone balancing treatment you will need to help treat your endo.

PMS A (A for anxiety)

This type of PMS is thought to be related to a relative oestrogen/progesterone imbalance, with a relative excess of oestrogen and a relative deficiency of progesterone, possibly related to poor liver clearance of oestrogens, abnormal progesterone production or faulty progesterone receptors. There's more info on page 95 in the section Reducing Oestrogen. This is the most common hormone imbalance seen with endo.

Symptoms

- nervous tension
- irritability
- mood swings
- anxiety

Treatment

- You may be prescribed a herbal extract of *Vitex agnus castus* berries starting on the first day of the cycle and continuing for between three and six months.
- Vitamin B6: 100–200 milligrams, or vitamin B complex containing 50 milligrams of vitamin B6 for ten to 14 days before the period.
- Magnesium: 200–800 milligrams daily of elemental magnesium in the form of magnesium phosphate, aspartate, orotate or chelate.
- Nevines such as *Valeriana officinalis* (valerian), *Scutellaria laterifolia* (skull-cap), *Matricaria recutita* (chamomile) for anxiety.

- *Withania somnifera* for anxiety with exhaustion.
- *Anemone pulsatilla* tincture is especially useful for tension headache with nervousness, especially when combined with *Passiflora incarnata* (passionflower).
- *Betonica officinalis* (wood betony) is used for headache and extreme anxiety, especially in combination with *Scutellaria laterifolia* (skullcap).
- *Bupleurum falcatum*, *Paeonia lactiflora* and *Angelica sinensis* is a common combination used in Chinese medicine for irregular periods with premenstrual anxiety and irritability.
- Plant oestrogens in foods and herbs (more info on plant oestrogens, also known as phyto-oestrogens, is in the Self Care chapter, page 87).
- Herbal and dietary bitters to aid liver clearance of oestrogens.
- Restriction of dairy products and sugar.
- 'Natural' progesterone creams, claimed to be made from plants such as *Dioscorea villosa* (wild yam) are sometimes advocated for the treatment of PMS, but the jury is still out on whether they help.

PMS C (C for cravings)

PMS C rarely exists as a form of PMS in isolation and often comes with PMS A. It's linked to functional hypo-glycaemia which may be caused by a magnesium deficiency, a sugar-induced sensitivity to insulin, or an imbalance in prostaglandins.

Symptoms
- headache
- increased appetite
- fatigue
- craving for sweets
- palpitations
- dizziness or fainting

Treatment
Blood sugar
- Magnesium: 200-800 milligrams daily of elemental magnesium in the form of magnesium phosphate, aspartate, orotate or chelate.
- Small meals often.
- Restricted sugar and salt intake.
- Dietary and herbal bitters to regulate blood sugar metabolism.

See more about prostaglandins imbalance on page 71.

PMS D (D for depression)
This form of PMS is accompanied by depression and withdrawal and is thought to be related to relative oestrogen deficiency. The causes might include lower oestrogen production around the menopause; a depleted oestrogen pool caused by being too thin or eating too much fibre; blocked oestrogen receptors caused by high lead levels; or a progesterone level which is relatively too high.

Symptoms

· depression
· crying
· insomnia
· forgetfulness
· confusion

Treatment

· Magnesium: 200–800 milligrams daily of elemental magnesium in the form of magnesium phosphate, aspartate, orotate or chelate, to decrease lead absorption and retention.
· Eat plant oestrogens, also known as phyto-oestrogens (see page 98 for more info).
· The 'oestrogenic herbs' which contain steroidal saponins such as *Chamaelirium luteum* (helionias), *Aletris farinosa* (true unicorn root), *Dioscorea villosa* (wild yam), as well as *Angelica sinensis* (Dang Gui) and *Paeonia lactiflora* (white peony).
· *Cimicifuga racemosa*, especially if you get premenstrual headaches.
· *Hypericum perforatum* and *Withania somnifera* for symptomatic treatment of depression.
· Coffee, alcohol, and chocolate aggravate feelings of depression, irritability and anxiety, as well as worsening many breast symptoms. Leave them alone during the premenstrual phase.

PMS H (H for hyperhydration)

PMS H is related to fluid retention thought to be brought about by an increase in the adrenal hormone, aldosterone, which is responsible for salt and water retention. This may be a response to lower progesterone secretion, too much oestrogen, magnesium deficiency, other hormone irregularities, or stress. Prolactin may be implicated when breast soreness is a big symptom.

Symptoms

- breast tenderness
- weight gain
- bloating
- swelling in lower body and eyelids

Treatment

- All treatments for PMS A and vitamin E: 100–600 IU daily, if breast tenderness is a problem.
- *Taraxacum officinale* leaf (dandelion leaf) as a tea is a mild diuretic and reduces fluid retention. Herbal diuretic tablets are also available.
- When fluid retention, bloating and weight gain are problems, usually PMS H, cut down on salt—most processed foods, including cheese, are high in salt. Also eat vegetables, grapefruit juice and bananas for potassium.

PMS P (P for pain)

In this category of PMS, the major problem is an increased sensitivity to pain which is believed to be caused by prostaglandins imbalance. Causes are thought to be elevated oestrogen levels, or eating too much animal fat.

Symptoms

- aches and pains
- period pain
- reduced pain threshold

Treatment

- Magnesium reduces sensitivity to pain in doses of 200–800 milligrams daily.
- Essential fatty acids such as evening primrose oil, 3 grams a day, with vitamin B6 and zinc, in doses prescribed by a practitioner.
- The herb *Tanacetum parthenium* (feverfew) is a prostaglandins-inhibitor and may help with period pain and migraine headaches if taken long term.
- If you have breast soreness, muscle or joint pains or period pain consistent with PMS P you'll probably respond well to reducing animal fats, processed vegetable oils, coconut, and increasing essential fatty acids and vitamin E. (Essential fatty acids are explained on page 120.)

REDUCING OESTROGEN

Too much oestrogen causes PMS-type symptoms and the extra production of endometrium (meaning there's more to go astray in an endometriosis sort of way). Oestrogen levels are influenced by a range of factors, including 'competitive inhibition' with plant oestrogens, and dietary changes and exercise to improve oestrogen clearance.

The natural therapist's aim is to keep oestrogen within normal limits, rather than reduce the levels below normal—the aim of some medical treatments such as GnRH agonists.

Oestrogen excess does not happen just because the ovaries make too much oestrogen. Many of us are relatively overexposed to the stimulatory effects of oestrogen simply because we are not making enough progesterone (see PMS A, page 75). The modern lifestyle (you party animal) also seems to slow down the usual process of getting rid of excess oestrogen through the liver and bowel, and to favour higher circulating levels of available oestrogen. Levels of oestrogen that stay too high seem to be significant risks for diseases.

The environmental oestrogens are introduced into the body from outside, mostly through food and water, and can also stimulate cells in much the same way as the oestrogens made in the body.

Symptoms

Heavier than usual periods, longer than usual periods, and PMS. Oestrogen excess is not only linked to endometriosis, but also fibroids, fibrocystic breast disease, breast and endometrial cancer.

81

Diagnosis

Excessively high levels of oestrogen are comparative to the levels of other hormones and so excess oestrogen cannot be detected on a single blood test for the oestrogen level. It's usually diagnosed by the symptoms.

Possible causes

Women who eat more fat have significantly higher blood levels of oestrogen. Reducing fat intake leads to lower oestrogen levels. A high fat intake has been linked with benign breast disease, breast cancer, heavy periods, endometriosis and fibroids.

Obesity can cause high oestrogen levels and can even interfere with ovulation. The more fat cells you have, the more fat cells the body has to convert androgens into oestrogens. This can lead to a higher risk of breast cancer, fibroids, and endometriosis.

Obesity is not just being overweight or carrying a few extra kilos. Women at increased risk are substantially over-weight and are in the highest range of the Body Mass Index. One of the ways to tell if body weight is within the normal range for your height is to calculate your Body Mass Index (BMI). You need to divide your weight in kilograms by your height in centimetres squared. For example, if you weigh 52 kilos and your height is 1.7 metres, you divide the weight (52) by the square of your height (1.7 times 1.7 is 2.89). The answer to the calculation is 17.99. Rounded up to the nearest full number, your BMI is 18, and that puts you in the underweight category.

Roughly speaking, on the BMI scale:

Less than 20 is considered to be underweight.

20–25 is normal.

26–30 is overweight.

Over 30 is considered to be obese.

But remember that the BMI is only a guide, and if your body frame is very slight or very large, give yourself a bit of latitude. (You know the phrase, 'Big-boned girl'? This is where it comes in handy.) And don't forget that calculating your BMI means nothing at all until you've gained full height—and that's always after you're 18 to 20 years old.

If you are very overweight, make sure your doctor considers the possibility that you have polycystic ovaries. This is a condition in which your ovaries make too many follicles and get out of whack and is associated with being overweight and some male characteristics such as excess hairiness.

Most of the natural treatments for excess oestrogen are self-imposed, so see the self care solutions on page 95. Liver herbs and herbs that behave as competitive inhibitors to oestrogen are also helpful. But they must be prescribed by a specifically trained herbalist.

You may not respond properly to dietary or herbal manipulation of oestrogen. Some people's hormones are so feral you can't kick-start them back to right levels without drugs. If you're one of these people, start with the drugs— you may be able to come off them later. You can do all of the other natural therapy treatments except for taking specific herbal remedies for hormone regulation. You can't start that until you come off the hormone drugs.

DEPRESSION AND MOOD SWINGS

If you're trying to get pregnant or might be pregnant, you need to be very careful of anything you take to improve your mood, whether it's drugs or something natural. Common herbs for depression include *Withania somnifera*, and some of the ginsengs. *Passiflora incatnata* (passionflower) and *Scutellaria laterifolia* (skullcap) can be used for anxiety. Any of these or other herbs must be prescribed by a qualified herbalist who knows you may be or may become pregnant.

ADHESIONS

Vitamin E is great for reducing the formation of adhesions. Doses of 500–1000 International Units (IU) of vitamine E each day can be used to prevent adhesion formation, although doses at this level should be supervised. If you're about to have an operation or you've just had one, give the large doses of vitamin E (more than 500 IU) a miss for a while, because there's a slight chance it will encourage unscheduled bleeding.

IMMUNE SYSTEM IRREGULARITIES

Calendula officinalis is a good herb to normalise the immune system. It stops muscle spasm, reduces period bleeding, as well as reducing inflammation. It is useful when there is dull, congestive pain with heavy bleeding; and in any case of period disorder with altered immune function. (All of these factors are common to endo.)

FERTILITY

Ovulation problems

In endo, ovulation can be delayed or the egg might not develop normally in the follicular phase. Or, you can develop luteinised unruptured follicle syndrome, in which the follicle develops but the egg isn't 'expelled' from the ovary. This is often linked to lower than normal progesterone levels. All these conditions are associated with infertility caused by an ovulation problem or early miscarriage.

Chamaelirium luteum (helonias) is known as a herb to regulate ovarian function during the follicular phase. It is used for ovarian cysts and for infertility. This herb is almost extinct now and its use is restricted. Other herbs can be used that have a similar effect such as *Dioscorea villosa* (wild yam), *Asparagus racemosa* (Shatavari) or *Tribulus terrestris* (tribulus). *Vitex agnus castus* is also useful for infertility caused by not ovulating, and for problems of the luteal phase. It is a difficult herb to use, and like others mentioned, should never be self-prescribed because it can overstimulate ovarian follicles. You could end up with having all your eggs in one basket, so to speak.

Other herbs known to enhance fertility, although exactly why is unknown, include *Aletris farinosa* (true unicorn root) and *Angelica sinensis* (Dang Gui).

General advice

Read the medical section on fertility on page 43. Some people who are still infertile after medical treatments will

85

try natural therapy as a last resort: others try natural therapies in tandem with medical treatments. All of the problems of endo-related infertility need to be treated to provide the most stable environment for conception to take place. They include prostaglandins imbalance, luteinised unruptured follicle syndrome, failed ovarian follicle development, infrequent ovulation, immune dysfunction and especially adhesions. Also, you'll probably need to have sex at some point.

Fish oils, star flower oil and evening primrose oil alter prostaglandins and leukotriene levels and may be capable of improving fertility. Evening primrose, from between 2 and 4 grams daily, and/or fish oils also between 2 and 4 grams daily, can be taken as supplements. A natural therapist will also prescribe herbs and supplements to improve ovulation regularity and hormone balance. Herbs for improving ovulation regulation and hormone balance generally should not be used if you're on IVF drugs unless 1. both your IVF doctor and your natural therapist know exactly what the other is doing, and 2. your natural therapist has had a great deal of experience using herbs and drugs together . . . this is a very tricky and evolving matter—needless to say, self-prescribing is out of the question.

See the Self Care and Eating for Health chapters suggestions on healthy eating and lifestyle for creating optimum conditions for fertility. Improving fertility can be a complicated and frustrating business—sometimes, it is not possible. The best approach is to combine specialist medical advice with natural therapies and self care. That way, you know you have done everything you can. Books on fertility are found in the What Now? chapter.

Self Care

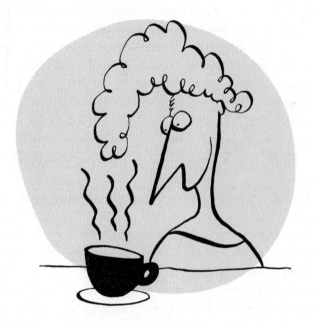

Here's a whole lot of stuff that you can do on your own to improve symptoms.

PAIN

- Cut down on animal fats (especially meat, pork, fatty cheeses, egg yolk and prawns/shrimps) and increase essential fatty acids in foods. The oil of evening primrose and especially fish oils can improve period pain.

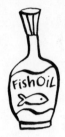

Usually a dose of 3 grams a day of either in capsule form is necessary to achieve good results. For the first few months, taking the supplements daily is a good idea. The dose can be reduced once pain control is achieved. Try fish oils first. Essential fatty acids are explained in number 8 of the Top 20 Eating Hints in the Eating for Health chapter.

- Calcium and magnesium supplements will sometimes relieve period cramps. Follow the recommended dose on the label. Usually, a combination of calcium and magnesium together is best. (An info page on both is in the Minerals section of the Eating for Health chapter.)

- Relax: it helps you cope with pain. Guided imagery and meditation can be useful as well, if you're into that sort of thing. Guided imagery is when you imagine yourself to be free of pain—if that works, try imagining you've won the lottery.

- Make ginger tea: grate 2–4 centimetres of fresh root ginger, place in a stainless steel saucepan with one to two cups of water, cover and bring slowly to the boil. Keep covered and simmer for about ten minutes. Strain, add honey to taste and sip while still hot. If possible, also have a warm bath. Other herbs can be taken at the same time. Ginger also eases nausea and is useful for period pain accompanied by nausea and vomiting. Commercial tablets such Travel Calm (Blackmores), are quite useful for mild period pain.

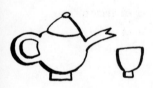

- A therapeutic massage just before or during the period can help. Some specific massage techniques like shiatsu, acupressure, and foot reflexology can be used to relieve pain, pelvic congestion and symptoms of hormone imbalance.
- Try aromatherapy. Clary sage, lavender, and chamomile oil are all useful for period pain because of their anti-spasmodic and relaxing properties. They can be used regularly in the bath, as a component of massage oil or as a warm compress, but should not be swallowed. These oils are not applied to the skin 'neat', and should be diluted with a base oil such as olive oil, or water.
- To make a massage oil, add between 1 and 3 millilitres, or 20 and 60 drops of each essential oil to 100 millilitres of a base oil (olive, almond or apricot kernel oil are good). Massage into the lower abdomen and back when pain is a problem. It may be useful to have a hot bath first, then use the massage oil. You may also find it useful to have the massage done by a large muscly fireman called Sven, who then slowly . . . I beg your pardon.
- You can make a hot compress by adding about 5 drops of each essential oil to a bowl of very hot water, soaking a cloth and then applying it to the painful area of the stomach after wringing out the excess water. The cloth can be repeatedly dipped in the water each time it cools. Alternatively, a hot-water bottle can be placed over the compress to keep it warm.
- An aromatherapy bath is easy. Usually only about 5–10 drops are needed in a full bathtub. Valerian oil can be very useful if the period pain prevents sleep, or when it is useful to 'sleep the pain off'. It can make some

people quite drowsy, so don't expect to be the life of the party afterwards. (Although we do know of a determined girly who used to take her hot-water bottle with her to the nightclubs and fill it up at the urn.)

- Heat of any sort will help to relieve muscle spasm. A hot-water bottle or a hot bath is cheap and easy. It is also possible to buy small hot packs that can be worn close to the skin—some manufacturers even sell them with specially made undies with a little pouch to hold the pack in place. ('Warmease' is the name of one product, but try a chemist before the sexy lingerie department.)

- Try a warm ginger pack on the lower abdomen. (It's kind of messy.) Place grated root ginger between several layers of cloth and place a hot-water bottle over the top. A little oil on the skin first will prevent burns from the ginger juice. Remove the pack if the skin starts to burn or sting.

  While warmth is helpful, getting cold can increase pain. Swimming in cold water can be a problem. The swimming itself can relieve pain, so go for a heated pool.

- If your period pain gets worse with exposure to cold, or better with heat, avoid iced drinks, ice cream or food straight from the fridge. Raw foods, like salads, can also be a problem, and raw vegies can bring on irritable bowel syndrome because the stomach has to work harder to digest them. Try warm food at room temperature or hotter; and add warming spices to food, like ginger, cardamom, coriander, turmeric and cinnamon.

- Having sex or an orgasm can sometimes help to reduce period pain by reducing muscle spasm and pelvic congestion. Hotsy totsy!

- There is a variety of ointments you can buy at pharmacies which are made of wild yam cream and other herbal extracts. We recommend that you give these a miss because research has not been able to validate the claimed effects. The creams are said to work because they contain herbs that regulate hormones, but there's no reason to rub it in rather than the easier and cheaper method of swallowing a herbal mixture or tablet. Last time we looked, the ointment price was about $45 and you're supposed to rub it into different parts of your body two to three times a day!

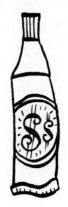

PMS

See the PMS section in Natural Therapy Solutions for extra self care hints. For severe PMS it is usually necessary to seek the guidance of a practitioner: most treatments for endometriosis will address your PMS anyway. Coffee, alcohol, and chocolate aggravate feelings of depression, irritability and anxiety, as well as worsening many breast symptoms. Leave them alone during the premenstrual phase. Women with PMS who use long slow distance exercise or yoga seem better at handling their PMS symptoms.

Getting light-headed and fainty between meals often aggravates PMS mood swings or depression, so if that's a problem, you may have functional hypoglaecaemia, which can be tackled with this diet:

Continuing functional hypoglycaemia diet

To be supervised by your health practitioner

When your symptoms have stopped, you can try coming off and following the Top 20 Eating Hints listed in the Eating for Health chapter.

Functional hypoglycaemia is caused by fluctuations in the blood sugar levels. Symptoms include fatigue, lethargy, sleepiness, insomnia, weakness, headache, bad moods, irritability, sugar cravings or unusual hunger. This syndrome is most likely to happen after stress, or the consumption of excess sugars and highly refined foods.

General guidelines

- Eat small amounts of protein regularly at meals and with snacks.
- Eat small meals often.
- Avoid all sugar, honey and dried fruit.
- Consume only small quantities of unsweet-ened, diluted fruit juice.
- Avoid all stimulants such as tea, coffee, choco-late, and cola drinks.
- Avoid alcohol and cigarettes.
- Eat wholegrain foods; avoid white flour and refined cereals.
- Always eat breakfast.

Protein

All animal protein is 'complete', and therefore meals containing milk products, eggs, meat or fish provide first class protein. Incomplete (plant) protein foods, however, need to be combined with complementary foods and eaten at the same meal to provide the same quality protein as animal protein.

Eat beans with grains: tofu (from soya beans) and rice; lentils and rice; corn and beans; buckwheat and tempeh; muesli and soya milk; kidney beans and barley. Or eat beans with seeds: tahini and beans; tofu and sesame seeds.

Or eat grains with nuts, nut butters on bread; rice and cashews; rice and peanut sauce.

Suggested menus

Breakfast

Choose from:

- Fruit with yoghurt, seeds and ground almonds.
- Wholegrain bread toast with nut butters, hommos or egg.
- Home-made muesli; oats, rolled barley, rice flakes, rice bran, seeds, coconut, and crushed almonds or cashews. Add fresh fruit and soya milk, low-fat milk or yoghurt as desired.
- Cooked cereal: oats (porridge), rice or buckwheat, with a selection of seeds.

93

Morning, Afternoon or Supper Snack

Choose from:

- A small handful of mixed seeds and nuts.
- Half a banana and a small handful of almonds.
- A glass of soya milk with seeds and nuts
- A small container of low-fat yoghurt.
- Two wholegrain dry biscuits with nut butters or hommos.
- Energy drink: Blend together half a cup of fresh fruit or juice, half a cup of low-fat yoghurt, and seeds with a small handful of almonds, and/or wheatgerm and lecithin.

Lunch

Choose from:

- Mixed vegetable salad with protein—either fish, cheese, hommos, meat or other appropriately combined vegetable proteins.
- Salad sandwich with protein as above.
- Vegetable soup with yoghurt, cheese, or a combination of beans and grains.
- One of the dinner choices.

Dinner

Choose from:

- Bean and grain dish: stir-fry vegies with rice and tofu; dhal with vegetables and rice; tortilla and beans; buckwheat noodles with vegetables and tempeh; vegetable soup with barley and red kidney beans.
- Grain and nut meal: steamed vegies with rice

and peanut sauce; stir-fry vegies with cashew nuts; pasta and pesto sauce.

- Beans and seeds: many of the Middle Eastern vegetarian meals are based on the principle of combined vegie proteins, like felafel and hommos.
- Meat or fish with plenty of vegies.

Eat smaller meals than you usually do, but eat more often: six half-size meals should be substituted for three normal-size meals.

REDUCING OESTROGEN

Endogenous oestrogens are the oestrogens made by your body. They help to stimulate endo growth, so they need to be dealt with to help treat your endo.

The ingestion of introduced chemicals, pesticides, hormones, plastics and preservatives in the food chain can also have an oestrogenic effect on the body similar to having too much oestrogen.

Natural ways to reduce oestrogen levels

- Eat less fat and refined carbohydrate.
- Eat more fibre. Natural fibre as part of whole food is recommended, rather than fibre-only breakfast cereals which provide no other wondrous nutrients. Eating more fibre can correct a blocked-up or farty bottom (known in the trade

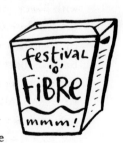

as bowel complaints), and reduce the incidence or severity of diabetes, gall stones and heart disease. A high-fibre diet lowers the risk rate of breast and colon cancer.

The best source of dietary fibre is from whole foods, but occasionally it may be necessary to use processed fibre products (like wheat bran, oat or rice bran), to effectively treat some diseases. Oat or rice bran, 'fibrous' vegetables (like celery and carrot), potato and other root vegies, tofu, legumes and linseed meal are all good sources of fibre if you have endo. Wheat bran may aggravate irritable bowel syndrome when it occurs with endo, and is usually best avoided.

The recommended daily intake for fibre is 30 grams for an adult from whole foods and not as fibre-only breakfast cereals. This could be achieved by eating the following in the one day: five serves of wholegrain or legume products (such as two slices of bread, a cup of cooked beans, a cup of brown rice, and a cup of breakfast cereal) and five serves of different vegetables and three pieces of fruit.

- Eat more cultured milk products and real yoghurt. Researchers found that eating these foods is associated with lower incidence of breast cancer which they attributed either to the reduced reabsorption of oestrogen or to other immune-enhancing effects of the lactobacillus bacteria.

- Eat more plant oestrogens, like soya products, ground linseeds and sprouted alfalfa. More on these plant oestrogens is to be found on page 98.

- Eat up the cabbage family. It helps break down oestrogens in the body. This includes green, purple and white cabbages, broccoli, brussels sprouts and radicchio.
- Look at your protein intake. Higher intakes of protein improve metabolism of oestrogen in the liver. Careful you don't overdo it—many other complaints are caused by excess protein. Try to get most of your protein from grains, legumes, fish and low-fat meat and keep it down to 60 grams a day. See the Top 20 Eating Hints in the Eating for Health chapter for more info on protein.
- Take vitamin B6. In vitamin B6 deficiency, tissues in the uterus and breast are more susceptible to the stimulating effects of oestrogen, and sadly, B6-deficient women with breast cancer have a poorer survival rate.
- Go easy on the grog. Moderate alcohol consumption (one glass of beer, one glass of wine or one shot of spirits daily) has been linked to a lower incidence of uterine cancer (particularly in overweight women); but an increased risk of breast cancer. If you have other risk factors for breast cancer it's probably best to cut right down on alcohol. Other women, including anyone with an increased risk of heart disease, can safely drink one to two standard glasses every second or third day. We don't really know what effect alcohol has on endo, but keeping your liver happy

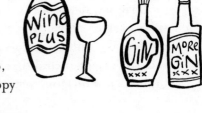

makes sense with this condition, so sadly, daiquiri binges are not recommended. Small and infrequent tippling is.

- Moderate exercise helps to reduce the production of oestrogen and increase its clearance from the body.
- Foods which help the liver break down oestrogen include beans, legumes, onions, and garlic. Bitter green leafy vegetables and bitter herbs prescribed by a herbalist will help liver function, which may help clear excess oestrogen.
- Reduce pesticide use in your home and garden and campaign for the same in your local area.
- Buy fresh, non-packaged food. (Fatty foods like cheeses, wrapped in cling wrap, can absorb oestrogen-like components from the plastics.)
- Buy foods packaged in glass rather than in plastic or polystyrene.
- Buy organic foods if you can, especially organically grown or range-fed meats.

Eat more foods containing phyto-oestrogens.
Huh? How come to reduce oestrogen levels, we are told to eat something called phyto-oestrogens, which supposedly are like oestrogens made by the body, but not as strong? Doesn't that mean we'll have MORE oestrogens? Well, no. It works like this:

Imagine that there is a restricted number of parking spaces for oestrogen in your body (these parking spaces are actually called oestrogen receptors, and they are on cells in places including the breasts, bone, uterus and brain). Now imagine that there are delivery vans bringing the oestrogen—some vans are bringing the stronger, body-made oestrogens produced by the ovaries. Some vans are carrying the weaker phyto-oestrogens you get from eating certain foods. If the phyto-oestrogen vans get to some of the parking spaces first, then the stronger, body-made oestrogens can't get a park. They circle the block, not being able to deliver their stronger, oestrogenic effects on your body.

(When the ovaries stop making the stronger oestrogens, as in menopause, some of the side effects of menopause can be avoided by getting in as much alternative oestrogen as possible, even if it creates a weaker effect than usual. That's why menopausal women eat phyto-oestrogens by the bucketful.)

We all seem to need the phyto-oestrogens to balance our levels of oestrogens produced in the body throughout life. There are a few types of useful phyto-oestrogens:

Isoflavones: especially soya beans and all other legumes; whole grains.

Coumestans: especially soya sprouts; and all other sprouted beans or legumes, split peas, mung beans.

Lignans: especially linseeds; and whole rye, buckwheat, millet, sesame and sunflower seeds, legumes and beans, whole grains.

Resorcylic acid lactones: oats, barley, rye, sesame seeds, wheat, and peas.

Steroidal saponins: especially real liquorice, and potato.

Increasing soya intake can be as easy as substituting low-fat soy milk for ordinary milk and using soya flour in cooking. Tofu is very useful, as are dried or 'fresh' soya beans which can be added to soups and bean dishes. If your supermarket is too Anglo for these, try an Asian grocery shop. Linseeds contain lignans and can be used in cooking or ground and added to muesli, porridge, or drinks, like a smoothie. They're also useful for battling the symptoms of irritable bowel syndrome, so they're a must in the endo girl's pantry. (The easiest way to grind seeds is in a coffee grinder you don't use for coffee beans. It's best to grind and eat them immediately so there's no chance of rancidity. Don't buy pre-ground linseeds.)

FERTILITY

Reduce stress, exercise, lose weight or gain weight if that is required, follow the healthy eating techniques starting on page 113, read the books on page 160 and seek professional advice early. Cut out coffee. Oh, and if recommended by a professional, have some sex.

DEPRESSION AND MOOD SWINGS

Try yoga, meditation and the stuff recommended below on stress management, exercise and healthy eating. AND STOP DRINKING COFFEE AND TAKING CRACK. Try out counsellors till you find a good one.

ADHESIONS

Adhesions are best tackled only with herbal or medical weapons. There's not much you can do on your own.

EXERCISE

Exercising often helps period pain, PMS symptoms, stress and depression, especially if you exercise first thing in the morning and it's of the 'long slow distance' variety. If you exercise rigorously during your period you may have an increased risk of endo, perhaps because it contributes to retrograde flow. Regular exercise can mean a reduced risk of endo because it probably reduces the rate of oestrogen production. So, don't throw yourself around quite so much during the period (and no hanging upside down from the monkey bars) but otherwise regular exercise probably won't hurt, and is likely to be a real help.

IRRITABLE BOWEL SYNDROME

Quite frankly there's nothing pleasant about having a grumpy bottom. Irritable bowel syndrome often accompanies endo, and can make period pain even worse. Because some of the symptoms of endo are so similar to irritable bowel syndrome, you mightn't realise you have bowel spasm instead of endo pain itself.

Endo and irritable bowel syndrome often happen together. Maybe this is because rogue prostaglandins can cause muscle spasm in both the bowel and the uterus, and it is also possible that the bowel reacts to the irritation in the pelvic cavity by going into a reflex spasm with the uterus. Maybe when one bit of the body goes into spasm, all the rest decide to go out on strike in sympathy. The following irritable bowel syndrome diet, and especially the seed breakfast, will help. The seed breakfast also has the advantages of being rich in trace minerals, calcium and the essential fatty acids which help to balance the prostaglandins. If the diet doesn't work, don't blame yourself; see a herbalist for stronger herbal treatment such as the anti-spasmodic *Viburnum*.

Continuing diet for irritable bowel syndrome

© copyright Ruth Trickey

To be supervised by your health practitioner

When your symptoms have stopped, you can try coming off and following the Top 20 Eating Hints listed in the Eating for Health chapter.

These dietary recommendations help to reduce the spasm, pain and bloating of irritable bowel syndrome, and to regulate bowel function.

Seed breakfast

The seed breakfast consists of a combination of seeds, pectin-containing fruit and yoghurt.

In summer
- Linseeds
- Almonds
- Pumpkin seeds
- Sesame seeds
- Sunflower seeds
- Rice bran

These seeds are ground daily (ground to a consistency of coarsely ground coffee) and then combined with the bran in quantities equal by weight. Any left-overs must always be refrigerated. Mix about 2 tablespoons of seed and bran mix with the following ingredients.

Plus, fruit:
- Grated raw apple *or*
- Stewed apple, pear or plums.

Plus, yoghurt:
- Plain, (unsweetened) low-fat yoghurt with live cultures (Jalna, Lesna, Hakea and Hellenic are all good brands.)

Throw it all in a bowl and dig in.

In winter
Cooked grains:
Add 2 tablespoons of the seed mix to porridge or rice and eat with warmed stewed fruit. Yoghurt can either be eaten with the fruit and grains or eaten as a side dish.

Herb tea
Melissa officinalis (lemon balm) *Matricaria recutita* (chamomile) and *Mentha piperita* (peppermint tea) in equal quantities are prepared as for ordinary tea (2 teaspoons per cup).
Dose: 1–2 cups between each meal.

Foods to avoid or reduce

- Stimulants such as tea, coffee and cola drinks.
- Cereals made from 100 per cent wheat bran.
- Fried food, pastry, cream and ice-cream.
- Breads and other foods with yeast.
- Refined sugar and foods containing refined sugars.
- Alcohol, especially beer and wine.

CONSTIPATION

Constipation is a common problem before a period. It aggravates period pain and slows down oestrogen clearance through the bowel. It is, in fact, a pain in the arse.

- Eat bitter green vegetables and dietary fibre and drink lots of water.
- Most laxatives bring on spasms of the bowel to push everything along, and this is exactly what you don't want, as a reflex spasm in all of the organs in the pelvic cavity can hurt like hell. You might need to take herbal extract mixture containing bitters to maintain regular bowel habits, but these should not contain any of the anthraquinone laxatives.
- Steer clear of painkillers with codeine: it often aggravates constipation.

BEATING STRESS

- Try the hypoglycaemic diet in this chapter which will improve many of your symptoms, and your ability to cope with long-term stress.
- Avoid stimulants such as coffee, alcohol, cigarettes, and wild affairs in the Bahamas.
- Adopt stress management techniques such as yoga, 'long slow distance' exercise, relaxation tapes or meditation. (If you're bored with the idea of meditation, anything that makes you have fun or feel relaxed will do, which is where a wild affair in the Bahamas might come in handy.)
- If your budget doesn't quite stretch to lust in the tropics, try herbal teas such as chamomile and lime flowers, which can be mixed together. Lemon balm tea is useful for stomach upsets caused by anxiety, especially when combined with chamomile tea.
- Eat oats or porridge, it's good for the nervous system.
- Rub a little oil of ylang ylang or lavender on your temples to reduce anxiety. Some people find these oils useful for tension headaches. You can also use a few drops in an atmospheric oil burner floating on water, or in the bath (Whatever you do, don't swallow essential oils.) For a list of oils that are safe in pregnancy see *Up the Duff* by Kaz Cooke.
- Rescue Remedy, a Bach flower essence available from health food shops and most natural therapists, is useful to relieve anxiety caused by one-off worrying events

like exams or public speaking. It can also be used for sleeplessness caused by worry.

IMPROVING SLEEP

This is a three-parter: dealing with the ease with which you get to sleep, the quality of the sleep and the time you wake up. Waking up too early, such as five o'clock every morning, can be a sign of depression and indicate a need for professional help.

- Cut out stimulating activities such as strenuous exercise or watching Alfred Hitchcock movies just before bed.
- Cut down or give up stimulants such as caffeine and sugar.
- Set up a relaxing bed-time routine such as having a lavender-scented bath and a warm drink like soya or cow's milk with honey.
- Establish a regular routine by going to bed at the same time.
- Go early. Many of the eastern traditions suggest that the two hours before midnight are the two most valuable hours of sleep to have.
- Avoid chemical sleeping tablets. Try over-the-counter herbal sleeping tablets, such as Nutricare's Kalms, which contain small amounts of valerian and other herbs that improve relaxation and shorten the length of time it takes to get to sleep. Because these tablets contain so little of the herb valerian, they do not cause drowsiness or fogginess in the head the next day.

- Too much vitamin B, especially B6, can cause wild dreams or nightmares. If you take vitamin B, take it in the mornings.
- If nothing works, get professional help.

THE 'GET PREGNANT AND BREASTFEED' SO-CALLED REST CURE

In societies in which women have fewer periods, and especially in the past, endometriosis was not often diagnosed. One of the reasons for this is that women without access to contraception were often pregnant or breastfeeding for most of their reproductive years—so they had far fewer periods. But frankly, staying pregnant or breastfeeding between your teenage years and menopause isn't the most modern of solutions.

The only good reason for getting pregnant is wanting to have a child, not gambling on an endo cure. Full-term pregnancies statistically tend to decrease the risk of endo, but this certainly doesn't work for everyone. Many women who have had lots of kids still get endo. Of course while a woman is pregnant she is not having her period so 'fresh' endo deposits will not be created during that time. In the same way, breastfeeding can be useful in curbing endo, for those women who don't get their period while they're breastfeeding. Usually there is very little oestrogen about during breastfeeding, as the milk-making hormone, prolactin is dominating.

This is one of those supposed 'self care cures' casually suggested by some people which must seem ironically painful for women who would love to get pregnant but

can't because side effects of endo have made them infertile. In other words, this common suggestion has the
bonus of not only being useless, but infuriating. If it is
offered to you by a medical professional, and you slap
them, we shall appear at your trial in support of your
actions.

LOOK AFTER YOUR LIVER

To protect liver cells
- *Silybum marianum* (St Mary's thistle) seeds contain
  the most potent liver cell protective compounds known
  to exist. You can get it at the health food shop or
  chemist in pill form: follow the label's instructions.
- Anti-oxidants, such as vitamins A, E and C, betacarotene and selenium.
- *Phosphatidyl choline*, or lecithin, is a major component of healthy cell membranes. It protects liver cell
  membranes from damage from the continual attack of
  toxins and free radicals.

To improve detoxification
('Detoxing' is always best performed under the supervision of a reputable natural therapist, not someone who
believes in 'breatharianism', or fasting for days etc.)

- Specific herbs can improve liver enzyme activity such
  as *Silybum marianum* (St Mary's thistle) and
  Schizandra chinensis.
- Sulphur compounds found in cabbage family vegetables, garlic, and dandelion can induce enzyme

reactions in the liver which assist with detoxification. Brussels sprouts and cabbage, for example, can improve the breakdown and removal of some drugs.

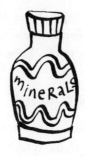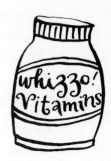

- An adequate protein intake is necessary to deal with some toxic materials.
- Carbohydrates assist with detoxification pathways. Low-kilojoule diets may not provide enough carbohydrate for the liver to function as an organ of detoxification.
- Minerals such as magnesium, calcium, zinc, copper and iron are essential components of many of the enzymes needed to drive detoxification pathways and are also involved in biochemical reactions which help to prevent free radical damage in liver cells. Information pages on magnesium, calcium, zinc and iron are in the minerals section of the Eating for Health chapter. Magnesium is a particularly good mineral because it helps with the symptoms of hormonal imbalance.
- Eat foods which help the liver correctly process oestrogens, especially methionine found in beans, eggs, onions and garlic.

To help your liver function, eat some of these foods when you can: endive, chicory, silverbeet, radicchio, outer leaves of cos lettuce, mustard greens, dandelion leaf, dandelion root ('coffee'), grapefruit, and any other bitter-tasting, green leafy, vegie-typey thingies. In the herbal department, look for extracts from St Mary's thistle, gentian, barberry, centaury, hops and artichoke leaves.

LOOK AFTER YOURSELF

Caring for yourself is not about self-diagnosis or treatment without proper guidance. It does involve learning to recognise signs and symptoms to prevent illness. If you learn more about your body it will help you to recognise early signs of any change that may need attention.

Here are some important things to remember about looking after yourself:

- Get tested. Breast exams and cervical screening (Pap tests) are available from local doctors, women's clinics and Family Planning centres. You should have an internal pelvic examination every year to detect any changes in the pelvic structures, particularly the ovaries.
- Learn to 'listen' to your body. This doesn't mean a hippy-drippy psychic version of the stethoscope, it means if you really feel like there's something wrong, there probably is. Don't ignore warning signs and symptoms.
- Take prescriptions from doctors and natural therapists exactly as recommended, and make sure that each of your health care providers knows what the other ones are doing.

- Don't self-diagnose, don't prescribe yourself drugs or herbs, and don't wear your underpants on your head.
- Be as well informed as possible about any condition or disease you are dealing with. Don't just read one book, or one theory, or listen to one piece of advice. It can be tempting to fasten onto one reason or theory to explain everything, because it's simple.
- Be willing to accept that self care can only go so far with some conditions, and further or more complex treatment may be necessary.
- Remember that even if you are doing all the right things with your diet and lifestyle, you may still need to manage an illness in other ways. Don't be mad at yourself, just think how much worse it would be if you had a packet of Peter Stuyvesants and a Coke for breakfast every day.

Eating for Health

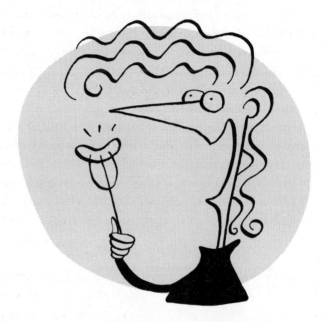

About the closest most doctors get to asking about your diet is to say 'Are you eating well?' To which you can reply, 'Oooh yes, doctor', meaning that you skip breakfast, have eight Tim Tams for lunch and usually eat the weight of a small Torana each evening, mostly from the food groups entitled 'lard' and 'utter crap'.

Natural therapists are more likely to pry into your eating habits and suggest some specific changes. Let's be frank: eating properly doesn't mean you'll never get sick, but it will make you healthier and less likely to get sick.

And it means you recover more quickly. Not that we're the type to say 'Oh, you've just had your leg amputated. Half a cup of dandelion tea a day and that'll grow right back in no time.'

There are also some specific foods and combinations of foods which can help with recognised conditions. That's why we included a couple of therapeutic short-term diets in the Self Care chapter. These are not like the short-term weight-loss diets and should be used under the supervision of your health practitioner.

Here's a 'top 20' of sensible suggestions for healthy eating. It's a general guide which you can use to introduce healthy changes to the way you eat. Don't try to change everything at once, don't regard the hints as a set of hard and fast rules and don't start faffing around the place weighing bits of food and stressing about whether you need another 76.4 grams of tofu before Thursday, or you'll bore yourself to death.

Remember that girls who haven't finished growing to their full height, and pregnant women, will need more of everything (well, you know, food, not bottles of gin) than the average adult woman.

TOP 20 EATING HINTS

1. Eat varied and interesting food

We're not talking about sitting down to a bowl of chaff three times a day with half a mung bean for morning tea. Don't eat foods you hate just because 'they're good for you'. Lots of different kinds of food is the go. And relax.

You're not going to explode if you have a chocolate bickie every now and then.

2. Drink plenty of fluids every day

Because otherwise you'll shrivel up like a dried apricot and blow away. Well, not quite. But you need at least 2 litres of water a day, and more when it's hot or you're exercising. By the time you have a dry mouth, dehydration has already started, so don't wait until you're really thirsty.

Fluids should be varied and should not come only from coffee, tea and fluffy duck cocktails. Two or three glasses of plain water, preferably filtered, throughout the day are essential. Fruit juices should be diluted because of their high sugar content.

3. Eat fresh and organic foods

Fresh is best—there are fewer preservatives, the food is less likely to be rancid, nutrient levels are higher and it tastes better. It's easier to see if fresh food has been spoiled or is old and past its 'use by' date. The closer you can get to the original source of the food, the better. This doesn't mean you have to go out and pick everything yourself, it means make sure your best pal is not the can-opener. Where possible, buy organic foods to minimise exposure to chemicals.

4. 'Therapeutic' diets are temporary

A therapeutic diet is prescribed with a particular goal—say, lowering cholesterol, improving anaemia, getting rid of thrush, or calming an irritable bowel. Therapeutic diets should only be used until the result is achieved, and always under the supervision of a health practitioner. Many of them don't contain the required nutrients, kilojoules or balance for extended use. If you react badly, go off it: therapeutic diets are not appropriate for all conditions or people.

5. Eat 5 to 7 different vegies and 3 fruits a day

Vegies and fruit contain a good range of vitamins, minerals, trace elements, essential fatty acids, antioxidants and fibre. Particular foods can also help to target particular problems. Cabbages and tomatoes reduce cancer risk; legumes contain plant oestrogens; bitter components flush the gall bladder; fruit pectin lowers cholesterol; and celery lowers blood pressure and reduces acid build-up in joints.

The old habit of 'a huge hunk of meat and three vegies boiled to death' should be abandoned with a sense of wild glee. To retain the most nutrients, it's best to cook vegies by steaming, stir-frying or baking. Every day you should eat from two to three different orange, red or yellow vegetables, a minimum of two green vegetables, and at least one of the cabbage family such as broccoli or cabbage—and some garlic or onion for their cancer-preventing and blood vessel protecting properties.

Fruit should be limited to three pieces a day because it doesn't seem to have the same energy-improving qualities of vegies (this may be because fruits are generally lower in minerals and higher in sugars). Fruit should preferably be eaten whole and not juiced, because juicing reduces the fibre content.

6. Main energy foods should be complex carbohydrates

Carbohydrates are energy foods which are eaten as whole foods like complex carbohydrates (such as brown instead of white rice) or as the more fatty and less useful refined carbohydrate like white bread. The main part of the diet should be based on complex carbohydrates from grains and legumes, dried beans and peas, nuts and seeds, soya products and some of the root vegies like potato, carrots and sweet potato. Common good energy foods include breakfast cereals and muesli, bread, rice, beans, tofu, pasta and potato.

Complex carbohydrates are high in fibre and many also contain plant oestrogens. They can lower blood cholesterol, stabilise blood sugar, regulate the bowel, reduce the appetite and ensure a good supply of regular energy. The slow energy release leads to greater stamina and fewer energy slumps. This is important for anyone troubled by blood sugar symptoms, and you there with premenstrual sugar cravings.

Carbo combos

Complex carbohydrates contain some of the amino acids which make up proteins and can be combined in a meal so that they become a substitute for animal protein.

 116

Carbohydrate-combining should be used by vegetarians to make sure that they get enough protein every day. The common combinations are:

- grains with beans: tofu and rice (Asia), lentils and rice (India), tortilla and beans (Mexico)
- grains and nuts: peanuts and rice (Southern Asia), nut butters and bread (bread-eating countries), rice and cashews (Asia)
- beans and seeds: sesame seed paste and beans (Middle East).

Many people instinctively cook like this or follow traditional recipes which incorporate food combinations. Combining carbohydrates gives all of the energy benefits of protein, as well as the positive benefits of complex carbohydrates without a high animal fat intake.

7. Eat enough fibre

Eating more fibre can help constipation and windy problems, and reduce the incidence or severity of diabetes, gall stones and heart disease.

The best source of dietary fibre is from whole foods, but occasionally it may be necessary to use processed fibre products (like wheat bran, oat or rice bran), to effectively treat some diseases. Wheat bran, 'fibrous' vegetables (like celery and carrot), potato and other root vegies, tofu, legumes and linseed meal are all good sources of fibre.

Fibre is sometimes included in therapeutic diets to achieve a specific outcome such as lowering of blood fats (cholesterol) and oestrogens; to reduce the incidence of gall bladder disease and colon cancer; for weight loss; or to treat constipation. Fibre is specifically important for women because it reduces the risk of oestrogen-dependent cancers, including breast cancer.

The recommended daily intake for fibre is 30 grams for an adult from whole foods and not as fibre-only breakfast cereals. This could be achieved by eating the following in the one day: five serves of wholegrain or legume products (such as two slices of bread, a cup of cooked beans, a cup of brown rice, and a cup of breakfast cereal) and five serves of different vegetables and three pieces of fruit.

8. Eat fewer 'bad fats' and more 'good fats'

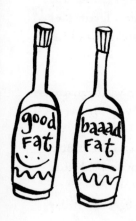

Fat is the devil! It causes heart disease! It turns you into a hideous gargoyle! You'll get cholesterol problems and your head will fall off! And now they've invented a synthetic oil with no absorbable fat which causes 'anal leakage'. So what! It hasn't got any fat! Hmmm. It's just an inkling, but maybe it's time to get a bit less hysterical.

The fact is that if you cut out all fats you'll have more problems than when you started. There's good ones and bad ones. We all need a reasonable level of fats in our diet. They are essential for the production of sex and adrenal hormones, for the health of our skin and mucous membranes. When the right fats are eaten, they protect against high cholesterol and heart disease, skin and period problems and a whole lot else.

Bad fats

- An overall reduction of all fats is good.
- Cut down on saturated fats—they're in animal products (pork, beef, dairy products and lamb) and in the tropical oils (coconut and palm oils). Excessive saturated fat intake is linked to heart disease, obesity and an increased risk of some cancers.
- Cut down on the Omega-6 polyunsaturated fats. High levels of Omega-6 polyunsaturated fats are found in cooking oils and margarine.
- Avoid trans-fatty acids. These are in oils which are processed to become solid, like margarine and vegetable shortening. The high temperature process changes the oil molecule, and destroys essential fatty acids ('good fats'). Trans-fatty acids interfere with the production of the useful group of prostaglandins which prevent PMS, period pain and a heap of inflammatory problems.
- Look for 'contains hydrogenated fats' on labels and avoid it.
- Overall, too many fats, sugars, alcohol or carbohydrates are converted into triglycerides which increase the risk of heart disease, kidney failure, high blood pressure and cancer.
- To reduce risk of heart disease, cholesterol-containing foods should be minimised, but the 'good fats' must be increased as well, to have the right effect. Cholesterol is used by the body to make hormones and other bits and pieces, so you shouldn't cut it out altogether. It is found in all animal fats but not vegetable fats. (The body makes its own cholesterol,

partly from eating cholesterol, and partly as a response to eating other saturated fats.)

Good fats
- To let the good fats do their work properly, you need to cut down on the bad fats, which can interfere with their work.
- Mono-unsaturated fats are the good vegetable oils to cook with and are more stable than polyunsaturated fats when they are exposed to heat, light or oxygen. Olive oil is the best-known mono-unsaturated oil and when used as a substitute for saturated fats, helps to lower cholesterol and reduce the risk of heart disease.
- Fatty acids are necessary for the normal function and development of most tissues including the kidney, liver, blood vessels, heart and brain. A deficiency leads to excessive scaliness of the skin, reduced growth rates and infertility in both males and females; and can also cause a greater susceptibility to infections, fragile red blood cells and difficulty in making prostaglandins.

Omega-3 fatty acids
The Omega-3 fatty acids are particular polyunsaturated fats. Suffice to say that we all need Omega-3 fatty acids, which are known as EPA (eicosapentaenoic acid), DHA (docosahexaenoic acid). ALA (alpha linolenic acid) is an essential fatty acid which the body cannot make itself from other fatty acids.

To keep your prostaglandins in balance, and to control imbalance-related conditions, like period pain, some kinds of infertility, wound healing—all sorts of things—

you need to regularly eat foods rich in Omega-3 fatty acids. To make the right prostaglandins, you need to include these Omega-3s in your diet:

Linseeds or linseed (flax seed) oil. These are very rich sources of ALA. You can take 1 to 2 tablespoons of ground linseeds a day. To help digestion and absorption, linseeds should be ground in a coffee grinder used only for seeds, never coffee (or mortar and pestle if you're feeling rustic), and can be sprinkled on muesli or tossed in a smoothie. They must be refrigerated in airtight containers or scoffed immediately after grinding. (Don't bother buying the pre-ground linseeds in packets at health food shops.) Alternatively, you could take 2 teaspoons of linseed/flax seed oil a day (to be refrigerated). When served as recommended, linseed oil has 60 per cent ALA.

Other sources. Pumpkin seeds (15 per cent ALA); canola oil (10 per cent); mustard seed oil (10 per cent); soya bean oil (7 to 9 per cent). Walnut oil also has moderate levels; and dark green leafy vegetables have small amounts. These fatty acids tend to go off and must be refrigerated in opaque bottles. No ALA oils should be cooked.

Oily fish. The best fish to eat are cold-water and oilier fish. Include some of these fish in at least four meals a week. 'Oily' fish are often deep sea fish, where they've needed a bit of protection from the cold.

If you can't buy fresh fish, get it in cans, although the benefits will be less obvious. Choose from: gemfish, blue mackerel, sea mullet, blue warehou, silver warehou, yellowtail kingfish, King George whiting, redfish, tuna, sardines, herring, pilchards, Atlantic salmon, silver trevally, luderick, ocean trout, blue eye, golden perch, blue grenadier, and rainbow trout.

Fish oil supplements are usually capsules which include 18 per cent EPA and 12 per cent DHA and are made from fish oils or fish liver oils. Cod liver and halibut liver oils, however, also contain vitamins A and D, which means that they are no good for the long term at large doses. (It's dangerous to take vitamin A supplements if you're pregnant.) Fish oils have a long list of therapeutic effects which includes reducing heart disease; reducing arthritic inflammation; and an improvement in allergy-related conditions such as asthma and eczema.

Omega-6 fatty acids
Linoleic acid. Eat some of this when you can. There may be positive effects on infertility linked to endometriosis and in reducing heavy periods. Linoleic acid is found in seed and vegetable oils, as well as most nuts, and organ meats. Coconut oil and dairy products contain very low levels of linoleic acid. Although the levels are low compared to seeds, any dark green vegetable is a source of linoleic acid. Linoleic acid is an essential fatty acid. Essential, in this case, merely means that you must eat them because the body won't manufacture them by itself.

There's lots of linoleic acid in seed oils: safflower oil (75 per cent); sunflower oil (60 to 70 per cent); walnut oil (60 per cent); corn oil (55 per cent); soya bean oil (50 per cent); peanut oil (35 per cent) and olive oil (8 per cent). They should be eaten uncooked.

Evening primrose oil, blackcurrant seed oil and borage seed oil are also rich sources of linoleic acid.

Gamma-linolenic acid. Gamma-linolenic acid (GLA) is the building block from which the body makes the prostaglandins that reduce inflammation, stop pain and activate the immune system. GLA is found in the oils of evening primrose, blackcurrant, safflower, sunflower, hemp, soybean, pumpkin seed, borage seed and walnut. These seed oils have been shown to reduce sore breasts and the severity of other PMS symptoms.

Evening primrose, star flower oil and blackcurrant seed oil are available as capsules which contain beneficial amounts of GLAs as well as linoleic acid.

Cooking and storing hints for oils

- Mono-unsaturated fats are the best oils for cooking. Pour them into a pan that's already hot to reduce heating time. Never re-use oils.
- Don't cook in other oils. Heating induces irreversible changes to many oils which leads to oxidation or free radical formation. Foods can be cooked in just a little water, or even 'dry fried' in a non-stick pan. Fish, eggs and vegetables can be poached in water, or a fruit

or vegetable puree and fish and vegetables can be baked rather than roasted in oil.

- Add oils to food after cooking as salad dressings or sauces.
- Eat more cold-pressed oils of linseed, safflower and canola as tablespoon doses once or twice a day or added to a seed breakfast or muesli, used in salad dressings, poured onto cooked food or mixed with yoghurt in a ratio of about one part oil to five parts yoghurt.
- Make your own spreads with avocado, tahini, yoghurt, chickpeas, nut butters or vegetable-based dips instead of margarine or butter.
- Buy oils manufactured without damage to the goodies ('cold-pressed', 'unrefined' or 'mechanically extracted') and in opaque glass bottles. All oils and oil-containing foods should be refrigerated. Otherwise they have a habit of going off.

9. Eat dairy products in moderation

Many people are sensitive to dairy products, or at least some aspects of them, and some natural therapists recommend that they not be eaten at all, while dietitians see the enormous potential for nutrients, especially calcium, and recommend a high intake. What's going on? Are they good for us or what? Well, they're okay, if you eat the low-fat varieties, unless you have a dairy intolerance, and even then, you probably can eat yoghurt.

Don't drink milk with lactose if you're intolerant. Here's a simple test: somebody comes up and asks you the time, do you strike them repeatedly with your handbag? That is very intolerant. (Seriously, any food intolerance or allergy should be appropriately diagnosed.)

Yoghurt is an important food. It is easily digestible, provides good bacteria which makes the gut work properly, has more calcium than milk, and may help to reduce the risk of breast and other oestrogen-dependent cancers. It is also well tolerated by those with a dairy or lactose intolerance.

Read the label to make sure a yoghurt has live cultures; many of the snack-type yoghurts don't, especially the flavoured and 'fruit yoghurts'. Get low-fat, no-sugar brands.

Don't forget bones need magnesium too, if calcium is to be properly retained, and dairy foods don't have much magnesium.

10. Eat phyto-oestrogens (see page 98 for details).

11. Eat enough protein regularly

When people go on 'healthy' or 'weight-loss' diets, they often drastically reduce or stop most of their protein intake. Protein is found in animal products such as meat, eggs, fish, milk and cheese, and also in the vegetable proteins such as tofu. Neither type is better or worse, unless you're a vegetarian.

Vegetarians (lacto-ovo), for example, can obtain protein from eating vegetable proteins, dairy products and eggs; vegans get it from eating combinations of vegetables. It's harder to get iron, and for the vegan, to get vitamin B12 as well. The advantage of being a vegetarian is a lower intake of fat and less likelihood of developing many of the chronic degenerative diseases; the disadvantage is a tendency to anaemia and fatigue.

Meat-eaters have an advantage when it comes to iron intake. Iron in meat is easier to absorb and it is present in much greater quantities. Animal protein is also of a better quality and meat-eaters can have a more relaxed attitude to nutrient intake and still maintain energy levels. On the down side, eating meat increases the intake of saturated fats and the risk of a number of diseases, such as heart disease and cancer. Deep sea fish is better because it contains high levels of essential fatty acids as well as protein. This means you have to ask the fishmonger if the fish is from the deep sea. Or there's a list of oily fish under Bad Fats and Good Fats, number 8 in this list.

For those who do eat meat, protein can come from (preferably chemical-free) lean, red meat in small quantities, some organic chicken without the skin, plenty of fish, no more than three eggs a week (also organic) and low-fat dairy products. You should have a combination of animal proteins and properly combined vegetable sources. How to combine them is explained in the hypoglycaemia diet on page 92.

It's kind of complicated, but on average, women over 20 should eat about 45–55 grams of protein each day. If you're between the ages of 11 and 20 you need to eat 1 gram of protein for every kilogram of your body weight.

Here are some levels of protein in food:

100 grams of meat	20–25 grams
100 grams of seafood	15–20 grams
1 cup beans/legumes	7.5–15 grams

1 cup whole grains	5–12 grams
1 cup milk or yoghurt	8 grams
1 egg	6 grams
30 grams of cheese	6–8 grams
1 cup vegies or fruit	2–4 grams

12. Know your minerals

The key ones for women are in the next section, astonishingly enough under the heading 'Minerals'.

13. Eat foods in season

Apart from the ludicrous price of foods that are out of season or imported (Darling, how marvellous! These July raspberries are only $6000 a punnet!) there's another reason to buy what's locally available at the right time of year.

All fruits and vegetables can be assigned with certain qualities in the same way that medicinal herbs are. Summer foods are generally juicy and light, winter foods tend to be dense and compact with lots of carbohydrate and protein. In summer, moist, easily digested raw foods make sense, but in winter they don't provide enough carbohydrate to counterbalance the energy expenditure needed to stay warm.

Winter foods should be mainly beans, legumes and root vegetables; salads can be made from root vegetables and cabbage. These are warming and comforting foods on a cold winter's day.

Most summer fruits and vegetables have cooling properties—melons are particularly cooling while bananas, which tend to be dense and compact, are warming. Eat stuff that seems instinctively right for that time of the year.

14. Vary the flavours

There are five main flavours in the diet: bitter, sweet, sour, salty and spicy or pungent. Australians traditionally rely heavily on the sweet and salty flavours, but other cultures include all or most of the flavours in their cooking as a matter of course—Thai food, for example, is cooked with the addition of salty, sweet, spicy and sour flavours. Each of the flavours has subtle effects on digestion and health.

Bitter

Bitter foods improve digestion and bowel function by stimulating the bile flow. Bitter green vegetables and radicchio, chicory, dandelion leaves and silverbeet are often included in the European diet to aid digestion. (Spinach is not a 'bitter' because it doesn't taste bitter.) Grapefruit is sour and bitter, and the old practice of having half a grapefruit before a fatty breakfast such as bacon and eggs makes a lot of sense. (Almost as much as not eating the fatty breakfast every morning.) Dandelion coffee is a gentle and effective bitter that is available as a beverage. (It is available as a beverage that tastes like bat wee, if you asked one of the authors of this book, but we shall draw a tactful veil over this fact.)

Spicy

Warming spices in the diet improve sluggish digestion and are particularly useful for complaints of the upper gastro-intestinal tract such as nausea, burping and indigestion. Ginger, cardamom, cumin and coriander are all useful—ginger tea is partic-

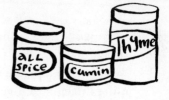

ularly helpful for nausea. (Cut two or three bits of fresh knobbly ginger root, about 2 centimetres long, throw them in a teapot, add boiling water and let it steep for a couple of minutes.) These spices can be brewed in ordinary black tea to assist with digestion. Warming spices are useful for those who feel cold, have difficulties with cold weather, or catch colds easily.

Sour
Sour foods are drying and can be used to stop snuffy noses. For some people, sweet foods cause phlegm or catarrh and sour foods can reverse the process. Many sour foods, such as citrus fruit, are useful to protect the mucous membranes from infections. Sour foods also aid digestion.

15. Don't stuff yourself silly
Overeating (to be perfectly obvious) is linked to obesity and a shorter life expectancy. The digestive tract is chronically overburdened and the incidence of gall bladder disease increases. The heart has to work harder and the risk of high blood pressure also increases.

16. Don't argue with your food
Eat foods which agree with you. Listen to your body and act accordingly. Some common diets cause obvious problems in some people, such as abdominal upsets, diarrhoea,

or fatigue. And sometimes your body decides it used to like something but now it's gone right off it. Raw food diets can be a problem, for example, because raw food is quite difficult to digest. Bloating, wind or even diarrhoea can lead to a depletion of nutrients and ill health. Trading one health problem (for example, shocking wind) for another (like being overweight) doesn't make sense.

17. Limit sugar and salt

Sugar
All types of sugar should be minimised, including brown and unrefined sugars; as well as the foods which are prepared with sugar and processed food with added sugar (this includes stuff like tinned beans, even).

Salt
Salt intake is associated with high blood pressure and increases the excretion of minerals in the urine. Most sodium (salt) enters the diet in manufactured foods, not through adding salt during cooking or at the table. Salt should be limited to around 3–5 grams daily.

18. Limit caffeine
Caffeine-containing drinks contain highly active substances known as xanthines. (Xanthines, while sounding like a girl-friend of Xena, Warrior Princess, are actually alkaloids which have diverse effects in the body.) Caffeine is in coffee, tea, cocoa and chocolate.

Caffeine increases anxiety, aggravates insomnia, helps to waste minerals and increases blood pressure.

Excessive caffeine intake is also linked with a number of common gynaecological conditions including endometriosis, fibroids, PMS and benign breast disease. Coffee has also been shown to lower fertility. Gynaecological problems have been associated with the equivalent of two cups of coffee or four cups of tea every day. 'Plunger' coffee has the least harmful effects. Boiled coffee should be completely avoided if there are problems with high cholesterol levels.

19. Cut down on alcohol

Women are more affected by alcohol for longer periods of time than men. Women have a lower body water content and so alcohol is less diluted. They also metabolise (break down) alcohol more slowly because they have a smaller liver cell mass than men.

This is why there are different government health warnings for women and men. Two standard alcoholic drinks in less than an hour will take a woman to the legal blood alcohol limit for driving, but this figure may be influenced by hormonal fluctuations of the menstrual cycle (around the period and ovulation, alcohol is thought to be metabolised more slowly), by cigarette smoking and by diet.

Excess alcohol consumption has been linked to cancers, hypertension, heart disease, foetal abnormalities, and liver disease. A host of other more subtle health problems are caused or aggravated by alcohol. Some are caused by depletion of minerals such as calcium, magnesium, potassium and zinc, and vitamins A, C and the B complex, especially B1. The National Health and Medical Research

Council have made the following recommendations for women:

- Women should limit drinking to two standard drinks or 20 grams of absolute alcohol per day and have two or three alcohol-free days a week to give the liver some recovery time.
- More than two drinks a day or 14 drinks a week is officially considered dangerous. Any more than that and you're officially damaging yourself.
- Don't drink at all if you're pregnant.

Also, if you do get legless drunk, don't go for the 'hair of the dog' and start all over again. Give your body free time to get over it: about two days between drinks is recommended.

20. Eat more serenely

A common cause of digestive problems and poor nutrient uptake, is the practice of eating in the car, watching TV or on the run. Meal times need to be a little sacred; a time set aside to think about food, be with family, friends or self. Taking time to chew food thoroughly is an essential beginning to good digestion. Avoid unnecessary argument or conflict and try not to eat when upset or in pain. If possible wait until you feel better. Most importantly, enjoy what you are eating. If you happen to eat some junk food, enjoy it, then get on with wholesome eating.

WHAT TO AIM TO EAT EVERY DAY

Don't thrash yourself with nettles if you don't eat perfectly every day. Here's what to aim for:

Vegies
A minimum of five different vegetables daily; from at least two green and two orange, yellow or red vegetables.

Fruit
Pieces from three different fresh, seasonal fruits.

Complex carbohydrates or whole grains and beans/legumes
Include four to five serves of grains such as wheat, rice, corn, hulled millet and/or beans such as chickpeas, lentils, red kidney beans, lima beans, soya beans and soya products. A serve is equivalent to a slice of bread, one cup of cooked grain or beans, or one medium-sized to large potato.

Yoghurt and cultured milks
Include at least one cup of low-fat yoghurt daily. If sensitive to cow's milk, include soya, goat's or sheep's yoghurt instead. Yoghurts should contain live cultures.

Fibre

Fibre should come from whole foods such as grains, nuts, seeds, fruit and vegetables and not from fibre-only bran-based, commercial breakfast cereals.

Fats and oils

Include three teaspoons of raw seed/oils in the diet daily, such as flax, canola, safflower or sunflower, but try to avoid margarine. To make 'better butter' mix equal quantities by weight of a good quality canola oil and butter. Keep refrigerated.

Seeds and nuts

Seeds: linseeds, sesame seeds, sunflower seeds, pumpkin seeds.

Nuts: almonds, hazelnuts, walnuts, pecans, cashews, pine nuts and peanuts.

Nuts and seeds have a high ratio of oils and should be kept to a maximum of half a cup a day. This should be substituted for one of the grain or bean servings, as well as one of the teaspoons of oil.

Protein

Protein is found in meat, fish, eggs, dairy products and properly combined vegetable proteins. Some protein should be taken with every meal.

MEAL SUGGESTIONS

Morning kick-start

Start the day with one of these:

- The juice of a lemon diluted in a glass of warm water.
- Half a grapefruit.
- Citrus juice.
- A whole piece of fruit.

(We're not suggesting that's your whole breakfast, but have one of them before anything else. It will wake up your digestive process.)

Breakfast ideas

- Home-made muesli: raw oatmeal, rice flakes, puffed millet, sunflower seeds, linseeds, sultanas, chopped almonds or cashews, dried pawpaw, coconut and chopped pumpkin seeds. Add low-fat cow's milk, yoghurt or soya milk, and chopped fresh fruit.
- Fresh fruit in season with yoghurt and seeds or chopped nuts.
- Wholegrain bread, toasted with nut butter, hommos, low-fat cheese, miso, alfalfa or other sprouts. You don't need butter with these spreads. Avoid honey and jams.
- Cooked cereal such as oatmeal, millet meal, brown rice or buckwheat, with added seeds or soya grits. Add milk of choice and fruit or a bit of honey.
- Energy drink: blend together low-fat yoghurt with either fresh fruit of your choice or fruit juice (about half and half), and add a teaspoon each of rice bran,

ground linseeds, almond meal, wheatgerm, and sunflower seeds.

Lunch ideas

- Wholegrain bread sandwich with a mixture of salad vegies. Include a bit of protein such as tuna, salmon, egg, low-fat cheese, or hommos.
- Salad of mixed vegies such as lettuce salad, coleslaw, tabouli salad, grated beetroot, tomatoes, carrot or celery. Protein should be included either in the form of correctly combined vegetable proteins or animal proteins as above.
- Soup with the addition of beans and grains, a little yoghurt or parmesan cheese.
- Any of the dinner choices or the breakfast energy drink.

Dinner ideas

Dinner should contain at least five different vegies, cooked or raw depending on season and preference; some protein; and a serve of complex carbohydrate like rice, root vegies, beans, or pasta. To keep animal protein to a minimum, combine meat with grain or bean dishes. Examples might be lamb and chickpea casserole, or similar combination, common in the Middle East and the south-eastern European countries; pasta and tomato sauce with tuna; stir-fry vegetables with a little meat, and served with rice, common in Asia. Or:

- Steamed vegetables with rice and tofu.
- Stir-fry beef and vegetables with rice.

- Steamed vegetables with lentils and rice.
- Grilled or baked fish with vegetables or salad.
- Minestrone soup with beans and parmesan cheese.

Fluids

- Limit caffeine-containing beverages to two cups of coffee or four cups of tea (and you know that doesn't mean you can have two megajolt triple caffeine-screaming long blacks).
- Drink at least 2 litres of water daily.

EATING FOR HEALING

In the past decade, the belief that diet can improve health and reduce the risk of a number of serious diseases has become proven fact. In particular, a low-fat diet reduces the risk of cancer and heart disease. And a diet high in fibre and plant oestrogens is likely to reduce your risk of getting oestrogen-dependent cancers such as breast cancer. Short-term therapeutic diets can be designed with a specific outcome in mind like getting rid of a complaint, or long-term diets might have a preventative focus. A diet might be designed around a specific life event such as breastfeeding, becoming menopausal or needing surgery.

Therapeutic diets

Be sure to get a professional diagnosis before trying any therapeutic diets designed for specific complaints, such as Ruth's special irritable bowel syndrome diet and hypo-glycaemia diet in this book. This is a serious business and you don't want to go faffing about with de-tox diets or the like without knowing exactly what you want to achieve and why. Stop when you get the required result.

MINERALS

It is better to get all minerals from food, but if this isn't possible (as opposed to just inconvenient) you can take supplements. Always check with your health practitioner for acceptable doses for you.

Zinc
Most women don't get enough zinc— especially during the teenage years.

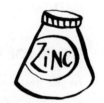

Some possible symptoms of zinc deficiency
Slow growth; infertility/delayed sexual maturation; hair loss; skin conditions of various kinds; diarrhoea; immune deficiencies; behavioural and sleep disturbances; night blindness; impaired taste and smell; white spots on finger-nails; delayed wound healing; post-op complications; dandruff; impaired glucose tolerance; connective tissue disease; reduced appetite.

Zinc deficiency can be caused by
Anorexia nervosa, fad diets, 'weight-loss' diets; exclusion diets for food allergies; a strict vegetarian diet; restricted protein diets; long-term intravenous therapy or tube feeding through the nose; alcoholism.

Zinc absorption may be hampered by
High-fibre diets; iron tablets; coeliac disease (gluten intolerance); food allergies; low or absent gastric acid levels; alcoholic cirrhosis; a dicky pancreas.

You need extra zinc if you're

- going through puberty or a growth spurt;
- pregnant or breastfeeding;
- taking diuretics;
- on the drug penicillamine, a detoxifying drug;
- suffering from psoriasis, exfoliative dermatitis, or excessive sweating;
- troubled by intestinal parasites or hookworm;
- drinking too much grog;
- suffering from liver disease including viral hepatitis;
- prone to chronic diarrhoea and ileostomy fluid loss;
- recovering from surgery or trauma;
- diagnosed with cancer.

Recommended daily allowance
12–15 milligrams a day for women.

Good sources of zinc

This chart shows how many milligrams of zinc in 100 grams of food:

Fresh oysters (as if you'd be having those everyday)	45–75	Peanuts	3
		Sardines	3
Dark chicken meat	2.85	Hazelnuts	3.5
Wheat bran	16	Walnuts	2.25
Wheat germ	13	Wholewheat bread	1.65
Dried ginger root	7	Prawns	1.15
Brazil nuts	7	Whole egg	1.10
Red meats	4.5–8.5	Non-fat cow milk	0.75
Parmesan cheese	4	Porridge	0.5
Dried peas	4	Raw carrots	0.5

Iron

Iron requirements for women are around 80 per cent higher than for men. It is estimated that iron deficiency is the most common nutritional disease worldwide and that more than half of all women consume less than the recommended amount of 10–15 milligrams a day.

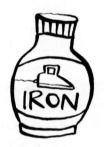

Those at most risk of iron deficiency

Pregnant women; women with heavy periods; children; vegetarians; serial dieters; people on strict exclusion diets; people with low gastric acid levels, such as after stomach surgery and with ageing; people with malnutrition.

Iron deficiency or anaemia?

Iron is stored in the body in red blood cells, the liver, bone marrow, spleen, muscles and in the serum. A test for anaemia will determine only whether there is a depletion of iron stored in the red blood cells (the haemoglobin level), but not whether iron levels are high enough in the rest of the body.

The symptoms of iron deficiency can happen before the red blood cells become depleted of iron. Many people are iron deficient even though their haemoglobin is normal. For this reason, many doctors now order a blood test to check iron stores in the plasma as well as the haemoglobin levels.

Symptoms of anaemia
Red blood cells need iron to be able to carry oxygen around the body. When that isn't around, anaemia symptoms happen, including poor stamina; shortness of breath on exertion; unreasonable limb fatigue and dizziness. Other symptoms seem to be related to the lack of iron in the serum, called iron deficiency.

Symptoms of iron deficiency
A red sore tongue and cracks in the corners of the mouth; excess hair loss; concave finger nails; reduced resistance to infection; poor digestion caused by low gastric acid levels. (Iron deficiency can cause decreased production of gastric acid and can be caused by it—a vicious circle.) Some people with iron deficiency have a strong desire to chew ice.

In children, symptoms include not thriving; slow learning; reduced infection resistance and poor appetite.

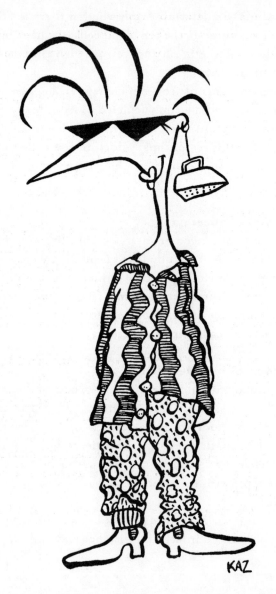

Iron is more important than ironing

How to improve iron absorption

Apart from increasing the amount of available iron in the diet, there are a number of other ways to increase iron levels:

- Eat vitamin C rich foods, particularly when consuming foods high in iron.
- Add acidic dressings, such as lemon juice and vinegar, to iron-rich foods. This is a common southern Mediterranean practice, where there is a high incidence of inherited anaemia and the traditional diet contains little red meat.
- Eat bitter vegetables or fruit before or during the meal to increase the flow of gastric acid which will in turn improve the absorption of minerals. Alcoholic aperitifs, grapefruit, Swedish bitters and bitter green vegetables can all be used. Bitter vegetables are best because they usually contain iron as well as stimulating its absorption.
- When low gastric acid levels are accompanied by iron deficiency, taking iron may improve both.
- Avoid tea (especially black tea) or coffee until the iron deficiency improves. The tannin in tea binds with iron making it difficult to absorb.
- Coffee also reduces absorption, especially if taken with or after a meal, but not when taken more than one hour before eating.
- Definitely don't take iron tablets with a cup of tea or coffee.

Diagnosing low iron stores

Iron deficiency causes the symptoms described above and should respond to a low-dose iron supplement within a few weeks. Iron should not be taken unnecessarily as it will accumulate in the body and may become toxic. If symptoms do not respond, seek advice and ask for a blood test which evaluates serum iron levels.

Recommended daily allowance

10–15 milligrams a day for women.

Good sources of iron

This chart shows how many milligrams of iron are in 100 grams of food.

Meat, fish and eggs

Mussels	7.7	Oysters	6.0
Lean beef	3.4	Lean lamb	2.7
Sardines	2.4	Eggs	2.0
Dark chicken meat	1.9	Lean pork	1.3
Light chicken meat	0.6	Cod	0.4

Grains

Special K	20.0	Wheat bran	12.9
AllBran	12.0	Wheat germ	10.0
Soyaflour	9.1	Weetbix	7.6
Raw oatmeal	4.1	Whole wheat flour	4.0
Rye biscuits	3.7	Whole wheat bread	2.5
White bread	1.7		

Legumes and vegetables

Raw parsley	8.0	Spinach	3.4
Silverbeet	3.0	Haricot beans	2.5
Lentils	2.4	Leeks	2.0
Spring onions	1.2	Peas	1.2
Broccoli	1.0	Raw mushrooms	1.0
Lettuce	0.9	Jacket potatoes	0.6

 144

Fruits

Dried peaches	6.8	Dried figs	4.2
Dried apricots	4.1	Prunes	2.9
Sultanas	1.8	Currants	1.8
Raisins	1.6	Dates	1.6
Avocado	1.5	Stewed prunes	1.4
Raspberries	1.2	Fresh apricots	0.4

Other

Yeast	20.0	Almonds	4.2
Brazil nuts	2.8	Walnuts	2.4
Peanuts	2.0	Hazelnuts	1.1

Magnesium

Magnesium is vital for the maintenance of bone density, the prevention of heart attacks and the functioning of all muscles. Magnesium is a crucial female mineral, but never seems to get the sexy telly ads, probably because calcium has a dairy corporation behind it, and the beef industry likes to bang on about iron.

Bones

Magnesium is almost as important for bone health as calcium. It improves the absorption of calcium from food and increases its retention in the body. A high intake of calcium inhibits the absorption of magnesium. Foods traditionally thought of as being useful for bone density, such as dairy products, are also relatively low in magnesium (a cup of milk contains 290 milligrams of calcium, but only 35 milligrams of magnesium) which raises doubts about the suitability of large intakes of dairy products for bone health. Magnesium, either alone or with calcium, offsets the usual overnight bone mineral loss.

The heart

Magnesium protects the heart muscle from getting overexcited which can cause irregularities in the heart beat.

PMS

Magnesium and vitamin B6 can help alter the hormone levels and protect against PMS.

Signs and symptoms of magnesium deficiency

Weakness and/or tiredness; poor muscle co-ordination; premenstrual symptoms; apathy; insomnia, hyperactivity; susceptibility to toxic effects of the drug digoxin; abnormalities of the heart's rhythm, an abnormal reading on an electrocardiograph (ECG) which traces heart activity; muscle cramps; grimaces, tremors of the tongue, 'flickering' eyelids; loss of appetite, nausea, constipation; confusion, disorientation and memory impairment, learning disabilities; vertigo; difficulty swallowing or throat constriction. Obviously these symptoms can have other serious causes, but when no obvious cause can be found, improved magnesium intake may help.

Recommended daily allowance

The recommended daily intake for magnesium is 400–800 milligrams for women.

Good sources of magnesium

This chart shows how many milligrams of magnesium in 100 grams of food:

Grains

Wheat bran*	520	Wheat germ	300
Whole wheat flour	140	Porridge	110
Muesli	100	Rye flour	92
White flour	36		

Seafood

Prawns	110

Vegetables

Beet tops	106	Silverbeet	65
Spinach	59	Raw parsley	52
Beans	35	Green peas	33
Broccoli	24	Beetroot	23

Beans and nuts

Brazil nuts	410	Soya flour	290
Almonds	260	Peanuts	180
Walnuts	130		

Fruits

Dried figs	92	Dried apricots	65
Avocado	30	Banana	20
Grapefruit juice	18		

---

* Foods that are rich in magnesium, such as bran, may not provide the best source of minerals. Magnesium can become bound to the phytates in bran which reduce absorption. Whole foods from a wide variety of sources is the best way to attain a good intake of easily absorbed magnesium.

Calcium

You can see below that the recommended daily allowance (RDA) varies depending on your age. If you are not getting enough calcium, you can either increase the number of calcium-rich foods, or take a supplement. To maintain the bone density to prevent osteoporosis you need to keep up a high calcium intake before, during and after the menopause. Post-menopausal women should consume 4–5 serves of calcium-rich foods in order to obtain enough calcium, preferably from different sources. In other words, don't just eat a vat of yoghurt every day.

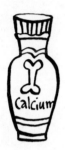

Recommended daily allowances
Babies: 350–550 milligrams
Kids aged 1 to 10: 800 milligrams
Teenagers: 1200 milligrams
Young women aged 20 to 35: 800–1000 milligrams
Pregnant/ breastfeeding women: 1500 milligrams
Women more than 35 years old: 1000 milligrams
After the menopause: 1500 milligrams.

Low-kilojoule calcium sources
Girls going through the growth spurt of their teenage years who are exercising regularly shouldn't worry about eating whole-fat dairy products. Others might like to consider these low-fat sources. All these low-kilojoule food sources have 300 milligrams of calcium:

1¼ cups of cooked spinach or other greens
2 cups cooked broccoli
1 cup Physical milk
⅔ cup plain low-fat yoghurt
¼ cup grated parmesan
50 grams Swiss or cheddar cheese
1½ cups whole milk
1¼ cups plain yoghurt
200 grams tofu
1 can sardines
300 grams tinned salmon
2 cups low-fat cottage cheese

Good sources of calcium

This chart shows how many milligrams of calcium are in 100 grams of food.

Dairy products

Skim milk powder (dry)	1190	Goat's milk	130
Whole milk powder (dry)	900	Skimmed cow's milk	123
Whey powder	645	Buttermilk	115
Physical milk 100 ml	205	Cow's milk whole	115
Yoghurt—cow's	180	Human milk	30
Rev milk 100 ml	150		

Cheese

Parmesan	1091	Camembert (30% fat)	600
Gruyere	1000	Danish Blue	580
Mozzarella	817	Blue (50% fat)	540
Cheddar	810	Camembert (60%fat)	400
Gouda	810	Fetta	353
Edam (30% fat)	800	Ricotta	223
Edam (45% fat)	678	Cottage (low-fat)	77
Gorgonzola	612	Cottage	67

Continued over page

Calcium sources continued

Eggs   56

Fish

Whitebait	860	Scallops	120
Sardines (canned)	550	Salmon (canned)	100

Soya products

Soya milk (dry)	330	Tofu	170
Soya grits	255	So Good soy milk	116
Dried soya beans	225	Vita Soy soy milk	32
Soya flour, full fat	210		

Nuts

Almonds	250	Walnuts	60
Brazil	180	Macadamia	50
Pistachio	136	Hazelnuts	45
Pecan	75	Peanut butter	35
Peanuts (fresh)	60	Cashews	30

Seeds

Unhulled sesame seeds	1160	Sunflower seeds	98
Linseeds	271	Pumpkin seeds	52
Hulled sesame seeds	110		

Grains and cereals

White flour	350	Wheat germ	69
Muesli (depends on brand)	200	Wheat crispbread	60
Wheat flour (white or brown)	150	Porridge	55
Wheat bran	110	Rye crispbread	50
Bread (brown or white)	100	Brown rice	33
All Bran	75	Weetbix	33
Rice bran	69		

Meat   10–20

Legumes (cooked)

Navy beans	95	Lentils	50
Chickpeas	70	Black-eyed beans	40
Kidney beans	70	Split peas	22

Sprouts

Alfalfa sprouts	28	Lentil sprouts	12
Mung bean sprouts	20		

Vegetables

Parsley	260	Onions	135
Watercress	190	Spinach	135
Dandelion greens	185	Broccoli	125
Spring onions	140	Silverbeet	115

Fruits

Dried figs	260	Rhubarb (stewed)	93
Lemons	110	Orange juice (100 ml)	60
Lemon juice (100 ml)	8	Blackberries	60
Other fruit except dried	10–50		

Other

Kelp	1095	Carob powder	355
Crude molasses	654	Brewers' yeast	210
Torula yeast	425		

What Now?

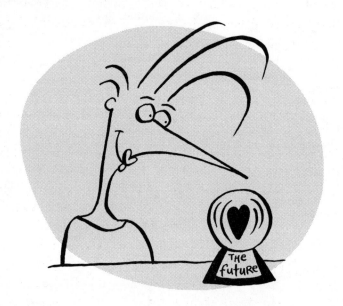

It's a tough, nasty illnesss, sometimes, this endo business. But now you know lots of ways to minimise pain and work towards a long-term solution that will be right for you as an individual. You don't have to call yourself a 'victim' or a 'sufferer' if you'd rather not. You can be a person 'with endo'. You don't have to call it a disease, if you'd prefer to say disorder, or even problem. There are many ways you can reduce its power over your life. But please don't try to do it alone. Friends and family will be able to be more supportive if they know exactly what it is—perhaps they can read this book too. And there is nothing like the comfort and strength of running with a pack—support groups can be fabulous sources of practical ideas, news of new treatments, understanding listeners and activism for more help from hospitals or governments. Welcome to the club, and congratulations for taking control of your own health.

MORE INFO

If your herbalist or naturopath wants to help but needs some pointers, they should get an up-to-date copy of *Women, Hormones and the Menstrual Cycle* by Ruth Trickey, published by Allen & Unwin, which has a comprehensive explanation of which herbs to use for various aspects of endometriosis treatment, and how to prescribe them.

Your herbalist should belong to the Natural Herbalists Association Australia (NHAA) telephone 02 9560 7077, or to the Australian Natural Therapists Association (ANTA), telephone 1800 817 577.

FINDING PRACTITIONERS AND SUPPORT GROUPS

You may be on the hunt for a good doctor, natural therapist, marriage counsellor (pain during sex can become a real problem) or other range of help for endo. You will find that some sites and resources are funded by drug or medical supply companies: this doesn't make the information necessarily suspect, it means that support groups are usually run on goodwill more than government money. Use your own judgement.

Here are some good places to start. The associations below are run by very organised, committed women who have had endometriosis themselves. If you're in a state or territory which doesn't have a well-resourced association, or seems to have gone AWOL, the Victorian group is recommended, and it keeps track of support groups nationwide.

Endometriosis Association of Victoria

This is Australia's premier endo group, staffed by dedicated women who've been through it all. There are special support groups for everyone, including young women. The association has a not-to-be-missed newsletter full of up-to-date medical info, and the way popular 'my story' section, soon to be released as a book. There are special events, and a really splendid library of specific articles, books and other useful resources to borrow or buy. They can give you names of specialist gynaecologists and naturopaths who treat endo. Becoming a member of this non-profit organisation will probably be one of the most positive things you ever do in your fight against endo.

Book

Explaining Endometriosis by Lorraine Henderson and Ros Wood—an update of this comprehensive book by two stalwarts of the Association, covering the emotional aspects of living with endo, how to get the most out of your doctors, and one of the most up-to-date medical sections you'll find in a book. (The book was published by Allen & Unwin at the end of 2000.)

Video
Endometriosis: The Inside Story—an American and an Australian woman have similar stories to tell which will interest anyone with endo. Contains treatment options.

Endometriosis Association of Victoria
28 Warrandyte Road
Ringwood VIC 3134
Phone 03 9879 2199, 1800 069 967 Fax 03 9879 6519
Email info@endometriois.org.au
Website www.endometriosis.org.au
The website has a popular glossary of medical terms.

Local support groups
There are many rural and remote support groups. Check with your closest 'Headquarters' below about finding one near you. Even if there's no state HQ near you listed here, do call one of those listed, as they may have contacts for a group very close to you. We haven't listed all the regional and suburban support groups here because they are often run by individuals, so the location and contact numbers change. The Victorian group usually has an up-to-date national list.

Endometriosis Association of NSW
All the above plus advice on access to specialist medical health care with both male and female gynaecologists who have a special interest in endometriosis, counselling access to a naturopath and nutritionist.
Hemsley House
20 Roslyn Street

Potts Point NSW 2011
Phone 02 9356 0450
Website www.pta.net.au/endo

Endometriosis Association of Queensland
This is accessed via a pager service. It will call you back with details of local support groups; regular get-togethers and guest speakers; treatment options; their library and resources, pamphlets including a glossary of medical terms. And its newsletter.
Wickham Terrace
Spring Hill QLD 4000
Phone 07 3836 3752

Tasmania
The Hobart Women's Health Centre has a library of endometriosis resources and a Menstrual Health and Endometriosis Information Kit which is free to individual women.
Hobart Women's Health Centre
326 Elizabeth Street
North Hobart TAS 7002
Phone 03 6231 3212
Email hwhc@trump.net.au
Website www.tased.edu.au/tasonline/hwhc/hwhc.htm

Elsewhere
At the time of publication it was hard to pin down groups in SA, WA or the ACT but keep checking the Victorian Association website or magazines or your local health department.

Clinics and hospitals
Many hospitals and clinics have their own support groups and libraries of resources related to endo. Your GP or local women's or public hospital should be able to put you in touch.

ECCA—Endometriosis Care Centres of Australia
A chain of private commercial clinics with range of practitoners, including surgeons, naturopaths, masseurs, and counsellors. Their library can furnish you with books, videos and tapes on endo and healthy lifestyles. The first clinic was opened at Clivedon Hill Private Hospital in Melbourne, and there are others in Brisbane and the Gold Coast and planned for other states. Each clinic has access to support groups.

Tape
Living Well with Endometriosis audio tape. Available through ECCA and sponsored by several drug companies. The tape contains an interview with a well-known surgeon in the area; a counsellor at ECCA and interviews with three women who have had endo.
Website <www.ecca.com.au>

Internet chatrooms
If you feel isolated and unable to get to a support group easily, why not try one on the World Wide Web? If you don't have access to the internet, call your local council or parliament member about a public access or community computer near you.

Use your search engine and type in variations of 'endometriosis chat' to find suggestions for chatrooms you can join.

WEBSITES

If you don't have access to the World Wide Web through a home computer, try your local library or internet cafe. (If you turn off the picture function, the downloading of words from a website will speed up and therefore be cheaper.)

www.endometriosis.org.au
Endometriosis Association of Victoria see page 154

www.nzendo.co.nz
New Zealand Endometriosis Foundation Inc.
Support group recommendations, resources, newsletters, and an education program for schools.

International websites are often quite small, covering a city area or affiliated with a hospital or clinic. They are often medical in emphasis. Here's a couple to start you off if you'd like to try a trawl.

www.endometriosisassn.org.
A Milwaulkee USA based site with book recommendations, and the usual explanations, resources, support groups etc. Affiliated with <www.ivf.com>

www.centerforendo.com
Centre for Endometriosis
Care North Atlanta Georgia.

www.awhn.org.au/home.htm
Australian Women's Health
Network
Women's health advocacy
network run by volunteers
which lobby the govern-
ment and try to post
important and useful links and
information on many women's health
subjects. Go to the Women's Health Issues link on
their home page and click on your area of interest.

www.mum.org
Museum of Menstruation and Women's Health
Okay, it's pretty weird that a guy has set this up and dedicated it to 'Mom' but it's full of amazing facts about the
history of periods, euphemisms, books about the subject,
practical and impractical products used to deal with
periods, attitudes through the ages and chat rooms.
Includes a page about the cats that live in the real museum
of menstruation in Washington DC, but a fun, if odd
visit, can be had on the net.

FERTILITY

Access Australia Infertility Network

Has a large range of contacts for counsellers, support groups and other helpful resources, including fact sheets on everything from coping with Christmas and other family holidays to polycystic ovarian disease.

PO Box 959
Parramatta NSW 2124
Phone 02 9670 2380
Fax 02 9670 2608
Email accessoz@ozemail.com.au
Website www.ozeail.com.au/-accessoz

Books

Battles with the Baby Gods by Amanda Gampson, Doubleday, Sydney, 1997. Personal stories from women with fertility problems.

Getting Pregnant: A Compassionate Resource to Overcoming Infertility by Professor Robert Jansen, Allen & Unwin, Sydney, 1997. A specialist in the field answers FAQs (frequently asked questions), with a reassuring bent. A look at medical tests and procedures you may encounter.

Pre conception self care

Planning a Baby: How to Prepare for a Healthy Pregnancy and Give Your Baby the Best Possible Start by Dr Sarah Brewster, Vermillion books, through Random House, Sydney, 1998. A medical perspective from England, including all sorts of recommendations for maximising your chances of conception, as well as how to conceive, and a section on the realities and sadness of miscarriage.

The Natural Way to Better Babies: Preconception Health Care for Prospective Parents by Francesca Naish and Janette Roberts, Random House, Sydney, 1996. Despite the unintentionally odd title (what makes a baby 'better'?) this offers ways to maximise your conception chances through good nutrition and lifestyle. Unfortunately, the suggestions to improve fertility will not work for everyone.

BOOKS

The Curse by Karen Houppert, Allen & Unwin, Sydney, 1999. An informative and political examination of how women are taught to be ashamed and secretive about periods. If you have a lot of trouble with periods you may quarrel with the 'periods are natural and wonderful' message but it's still a fascinating story about 'the last unmentionable taboo: menstruation' and the surprisingly long-lasting theme of 'feminine hygeine'. American.

Index

07/18/05